Between Jerusalem and Athens

Christian Explorations in Psychology
Edited by David G. Benner and Hendrika Vande Kemp

Between Jerusalem and Athens

Ethical Perspectives on Culture, Religion, and Psychotherapy

Alvin C. Dueck

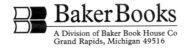
Baker Books

A Division of Baker Book House Co
Grand Rapids, Michigan 49516

Published by Baker Books
a division of Baker Book House Company
P.O. Box 6287, Grand Rapids, MI 49516-6287

Printed in the United States of America

Library of Congress Cataloging-in-Publication Data

Duek, Alvin C., 1943–
    Between Jerusalem and Athens: ethical perspectives on culture,
religion, and psychotherapy/Alvin C. Dueck.
        p. cm.—(Christian explorations in psychology)
    Includes bibliographical references and index.
    ISBN 0-8010-2008-5 (pbk.)
    1. Psychologists—Professional ethics. 2. Psychology—Moral and
ethical aspects. 3. Psychology and religion. 4. Psychology—Religious
aspects—Christianity. I. Title. II. Series.
BF76.4.D84 1995
174p.915—dc20   95-15357

Contents

Preface

The religious world is a composite of diverse communities. The larger religious community is enriched if each ethnoreligious group reflects on the issues of being a faithful Christian in society from its unique vantage point. This book emerges out of the lived experience of a Mennonite psychologist. I take particularity seriously. I do not attempt to create an overarching Christian psychology. Rather, I reflect on the issues facing the profession of psychotherapy from the perspective of my experience within one strand of Christianity. Although my experiences are read through the glasses of one who grew up in a Mennonite community, I nonetheless see myself as a world Christian.

As such I have been a member of many communities, all of which have shaped me. Those in my community who have shaped the conversations along the way between Athens and Jerusalem include other psychologists, pastors, theologians, sociologists, clients, friends, and fellow believers in all walks of life. I think specifically of professors John Quiring, Frank C. Peters, and Professor Robson, who first piqued my interest in psychology; John Toews, Stanley Hauerwas, Howard Loewen, Dena Pence-Frantz, Delbert Wiens, and John Howard Yoder, who helped me understand the theological contribution of the Believers' Church heritage; Robert Enns, Cal Redekop, and Paul Toews, who asked the larger sociological and historical questions; and Irene Loewen, Kirk Farnsworth, Vic Koop, Karl

Bartsch, Delores Friesen, Newton Maloney, John Friesen, Carolyn Holderread Heggen, Dave Augsburger, John Lee, Dean Kliewer, Brent Lindquist, Chris Rosik, Jan Ritchey, Siang Yan Tan, and Hendrika Vande Kemp, who nurtured my clinical perspectives. Over the years there have been students who assisted with research to whom I am grateful: Gordon Zerbe, Will Friesen, Mike Klassen, Adrian Block, Mike Regier, Kevin Genich, Katrina Poetker, Connie Enns-Rempel, Walter Thiessen, Phyllis Martens, David Fast and Colin Collett. The following journals and publishers have graciously permitted me the use of material I published earlier in their publications: Herald Press, *Conrad Grebel Review*, *Mennonite Quarterly Review*, Baker Book House, *Journal of Psychology and Theology*, *Journal of Psychology and Christianity*, and *Pastoral Psychology*. My bibliography references the many others who have influenced my thinking. (I might add that where authors did not use gender inclusive language when they are quoted, no changes were made.) I am grateful to the members of the Association of Mennonite Psychologists and members of the College Community Church, who have stimulated thought and provided critique. My clients have kept me honest and in contact with the reality my reflections point to. My wife, Anne, in her loving care for Alzheimer's adults, has continually modeled for me the way one integrates faith and profession. Our children have encouraged me by their commitment to incarnating the vision of the Reign of God in their marriages and their lives.

Spring 1995

Introduction: On Traveling between Jerusalem and Athens

What has Jerusalem to do with Athens? Tertullian's question still stands. What has the culture of Jerusalem to do with the culture of Athens?

Psychology is a discipline profoundly shaped by the culture of Hellenism, with its commitment to idealism, empiricism, humanism, and naturalism in psychological reflections. My spiritual heritage, however, is the culture of Jerusalem, with its stories of the creation of a people of God, with its community of Jesus' followers and the outpouring of the Spirit on individuals. Exodus, crucifixion and resurrection, and Pentecost are the critical events in this cultural narrative. These events, in the Jerusalem community, are the frame of reference for understanding Athens or modernity, the death of Socrates, or the Bill of Human Rights.

The ethos of Athens is different from that of Jerusalem. In Athens the gods are many, the epistemology articulate, the psychology explicit, and the culture cosmopolitan. In Jerusalem, there is little talk of epistemology or psychology and the culture is tribal and provincial. But there is much talk about Yahweh's justice, mercy, and convenantal faithfulness.

I live in both cultures. At times I feel like a resident alien carrying my cultural "green card" in Greek society; its stories, characters, and rituals seem foreign. On the other hand, my experience of living in ethnic Jerusalem has often been one of isolation, though here I have the familiarity of tradition, ritual, and kin.

I am a regular traveler on the road between Jerusalem and Athens, talking with other pilgrims about the psychologies of the two different cultures. The wayfarers I meet are fascinating. There are those eager to leave behind the restrictive provincialism of ethnic Judaism and Christianity and excited about encountering the cosmopolitanism of Hellenism. At the other extreme are those returning from Athens eager to rediscover their roots, tired of the uncertainty of relativism and pluralism.

When sojourning in Athens, I find colleagues who assume that Athens and Jerusalem are fundamentally identical in ethic and ethos. For them the psychology of being human is universal.

When in Jerusalem on retreat, I find professional psychologists chanting the language of their faith, assuming that anyone who has ears to hear will understand their particularity.

I find myself most intrigued with those pilgrims who are open to the ways God works in different cultures—Athenian, Babylonian, or Syrian; American, Russian, or Asian; premodern, modern, or postmodern. For them God is the God of Jew and of Gentile. The old stories of Abraham, Sarah, Moses, Miriam, Jesus, Mary, and Paul are the stories that shape their pilgrimage and sense of identity even in strange lands. They are not so provincial as to be unable to see God at work in cultures other than their own.

Maps, Creeds, and Codes

This is a book about ethics for professional psychologists. I am concerned about tension and continuity between the ethos of Jerusalem and that of Athens, between the ethic of the American mental health profession and that of Christianity, realizing that there is diversity in both. Our country, the various professions, and our religious culture all have implicit (ethos) and explicit (ethical) expectations for their members. What are the expectations that so powerfully shape professionals, citizens, and congregants? At issue is not *whether* we will be socialized by our social context, but *how*. The questions for therapists is not whether we are ethicists, but what kind of ethicists we are implicitly and what kind of ethical convictions we hold explicitly.

Culture is not ethically neutral, something that can simply be described in objective social science terminology. A culture pulsates with value and conviction. Culture managers, ancient or modern, assume that their members will reflect the primary values of the culture. The American public assumes that it is appropriate to expect of its members that their character reflect the basic values of the Constitution. Professional societies, such as the American Psychological Association, are institutions legitimated by American culture, and it is assumed that its members will support, at a fundamental level, treasured cultural values such as individual autonomy, privacy, and the freedom of speech. When culture and guilds establish expectations, then the individual professional becomes an ethical agent of that larger social context. In varying degrees, professionals mediate the values of the larger wholes—neighborhood, community, society, culture. To the extent that they reflect on which values are worth reinforcing, to that extent psychologists and therapists are ethicists and social agents.

The religious community is no different. Religious bodies anticipate that members who voluntarily join can be expected to share the community's most central convictions. It should come as no surprise that they also assume that these convictions would shape the behavior of their members in various life settings, including the professional setting.

Hoping to shape the ethical behavior of their adherents, national, religious, and professional communities issue ethical statements that outline expectations for their members. Societies enact laws, professions create codes, the church issues position papers. The purpose of ethical statements is to make public the values and beliefs that characterize the respective communities. The statements include those specific behaviors that each community assumes can be reasonably expected of individuals who call themselves members. In professions, those members who conform are considered ethical. In religious bodies, those who profoundly embody the ethic are considered saints. Those who reject a community's values, disregard its beliefs, or act inconsistently may experience the social sanctions of the community—they may be ignored, asked to change or to leave.

The ethical code for psychologists (APA, 1992) assumes both an ethos and an ethic. The attitudes (ethos) are supported by the assumptions of modern Western cultures: responsibility for the consequences of personal actions; commitment to free inquiry; honest self-presentation; tolerance of diversity of attitudes; accountability to colleagues, profession, and society; respect for the legislation designed to protect the disadvantaged; loyalty to the profession; respect for confidentiality. The ethic could include the following actions in a profession: recognition of the limitations of work; objective research and public presentation; competence in knowledge and skills; separation of professional and nonprofessional roles; avoidance of sexual or financial exploitation; altruism in services; recognition of one's interdependence with other professional resources; and the honoring of promises to subjects or clients.

The religious community also assumes an ethos and declares an ethic. The ethos of the Christian community may include openness and commitment to God as the source of personal life, hope for a society ordered by a consciousness of God, respect for humanity as made in the image of God, recognition of our interdependence in the human community, willingness to so live one's life as to be consistent with the example of Jesus. The behavioral manifestation of the religious ethos might also include involvement in the life of the Christian community, sexual fidelity, concern for the poor, willingness to share the story of faith, integrity in relationships, and fiscal honesty.

What Jerusalem and Athens do have in common is that they seek to create an ethic. Both tend to assume there is sufficient moral ethos in the larger culture to sustain their ethic. It is not, then, as if Christians must deal with ethical issues in their therapy but secularists do not. The critical issue for the religious psychotherapist is how to live with two ethical cultures.

Some might argue that after two millennia of conversation these two cultures are not as distinct as they once were. However, when I observe the current hiatus between religion and therapy, my sharp distinction between Athens and Jerusalem seems justified. When I examine again the ethical character of the Reign of God, the gap between Jerusalem and Athens widens. Nonetheless, it is in Athens that I reside, and I am called both to live with the tension and to transcend it.

The Psychotherapist as Ethicist:
Cartographer and Tour Guide

Why a book on ethics and therapy? First, the myth of the morally neutral therapist largely persists. The argument runs as follows: therapists do not impose ethical positions on clients—or so we are told. Therapists are technicians of change, not ethicists. They deal with psychological disorders, not personal values of health. Their discourse is that of therapy, not ethics. Since there is no rationally defensible hierarchy of values in a pluralist society, the therapist cannot advocate particular values. And to argue that culture is inherently ethical is irrelevant since the ethical therapist is loyal first and foremost to the client, not to the larger culture. If therapists are to be considered ethicists at all, they are the kind that build their practice on the basis of value-neutral science. They are scientist-practitioners.

Value neutrality is a myth that serves the socially amnesic professional. All therapists are ethical agents of some culture or community, whether they realize it or not (Tjeltveit, 1992). They are cartographers and tour guides for a better culture. The language of neutrality is quite appropriate if the term refers to emotional impartiality or rejection of coercion. But therapists *are* members of a culture and of communities, and as such implicitly possess values and convictions. Therapy is clearly a socializing process; it expects change. To set a therapeutic goal is to become an ethicist.

In the face of flagrant ethical violations, both churches and professions have frantically expanded their ethical codes to guarantee the ethical character of their members. But in the last analysis it is not pronouncements that will create the ethos necessary to sustain ethical character. Increasingly the question emerges whether *any* culture, secular or religious, Athens or Jerusalem, has the potential to create an ethos that reflects its ethic (MacIntyre, 1981). This book seeks to encourage religious professionals to reflect ethically on their work. Too often the church is seen simply as a sanctuary for the weak, an enclave for the faithful, or a setting for sermonizing. Rather, the church is a community of ethical discernment for professionals who seek to be ethical.

Ethics and "Integration": Traveling Together

Why focus on the role of ethics in the dialogue between religion and therapy? In religious circles we tend to neglect discussion of ethics in therapy. Efforts at relating psychology or psychotherapy to Christian concerns tend to remain abstract, and the concrete implications tend to be ignored, neglected, or simply appended. In the end, our research or therapy reflects business as usual.

This book seeks to make a contribution to the discussion of "integration," but from the perspective of theological ethics. Current attempts at "integration"—that is, traveling together—seem to be efforts directed at harmonizing the contradictory languages of two different cultures: Christianity and psychotherapy. It is assumed that there exist two coherent universes of moral discourse and that they must in some way be blended. Contemporary journals such as the *Journal of Psychology and Theology,* the *Journal of Religion and Health,* the *Journal of Pastoral Care, Pastoral Psychology, Journal of Psychology and Christianity, Journal of Psychology and Judaism,* and *Lumen Vitae* all assume that integrating religion and psychology is mutually beneficial. The religious cultures considered normative or ethically resourceful may vary in the journals (Jewish, Evangelical, Protestant, Catholic, etc.), but all assume a positive stance toward companionship along the way.

The term "integration," however, fails to indicate where the journey begins. The integrationist metaphor does not indicate whether the ethic implicit in modern psychology or that of Christianity is the starting point. There is no inherent priority for the starting point in the metaphor of integration. Hence, American ethnic minorities have become wary of talk of racial integration. It tends to mean assimilation. If American culture is dominant, then integration of Christianity and psychology most often means psychologizing Christianity in ways consistent with the moral vocabulary of the American psychologist. The assimilationist may well overestimate the available resources of contemporary religious or secular cultures, and underestimate the difference between the ethic of Jerusalem and of Athens.

So articles and books continue to be churned out that provide one more version of psychoanalyzed Christianity or one more declaration that the ideas of Jung are synonymous with that of Jesus. Grace and Rogerian unconditional acceptance, we are told, are truly identical. In each case the psychological concepts overdetermine the conversation in much the same way that questions and concepts of philosophical ethics have overdetermined Christian ethics in the past. In the process we distort both the discipline of psychology and the worldview of Christianity.

Sometimes in discussions about the relationship between the travel partners, I am left with the impression that if we repeat the buzzword "integration" enough, a relationship between the therapeutic community and the Christian community will magically appear. "Integration" as metaphor needs some serious reevaluation. First, one can only truly integrate a new culture when one has a sense of one's own personal identity. Second, how can one integrate two cultures that have increasingly less ability to shape the character of their own members? Third, integration means little if one is committed to monoculturalism, when integration means translating one discipline into the cultural language of the other. The metaphor "integration" does not take seriously a more critical perspective as the prerequisite for conversation between cultures. The dominant culture (American, Caucasian, male, middle class) often controls the nature of the dialogue.

Evangelical psychologists often assume that theory and practice occur beyond history. It is somehow assumed that the historical context in which we counsel and teach is irrelevant. When evangelicals "do integration," the model is very abstract. The integration that emerges is rationalistic in nature; it consists primarily of a systematic combination of ideas and insights from theology and the human sciences. What is not clear is whether this model of integration really makes a difference in practice. After we have more carefully examined the ethical resources available in American culture and psychology, the cultural exchange will be more appropriate and significant.

The Ethic of Jerusalem and the Reign of God

Perhaps the most important purpose of this book is to explore the theme of the Reign of God as a metaphor for guiding dialogue between culture, religion, and psychotherapy. One could begin with the image of God within, the nature of evil, or the role of atonement in therapy as the guiding theological theme. I have chosen the Reign of God as a theme because its implications for context and content of therapy are profound. It seems impossible to pursue this theme without it in some way affecting the form or setting of therapy. There are professional therapists for whom a religious perspective is a matter of Sunday worship and is irrelevant to the healing profession. Such compartmentalization seems foreign to the implicit wholism of the theme of the Reign of God.

Those who claim to be Christians and are trained in a helping profession must first decide where their primary loyalty and identity lies: Jerusalem or Athens. After all, how can one have two normative maps, codes, or confessions? I will begin with the ethos/ethic that a Christian therapist considers primary: the confession of the historic Christian community. We are invited to seek first the Reign of God (Matt. 6:33).

To say one's identity is Judeo-Christian doesn't preclude travel to and from Athens. Nor does it mean that upon arrival in Athens there is nothing for us to learn. It *does* mean that other cultures, communities, and therapies are interpreted from within the frame of a primary ethical commitment. Religious therapists assume that their faith story has clear implications for the way they view therapy, meaning, human identity, or tragedy.

For this reason, I will begin with a theme familiar to residents of Jerusalem: the Reign of God. This is, in fact, a central theme in the biblical tradition (Snyder, 1991; Kraybill, 1978). The Reign of God will serve to guide the reflections in each of the three sections of this book: culture, community, and character. The Reign of God can be incarnated, made explicit, in each of these three forms.

- As an ethical culture, the story of the Reign of God can provide the narrative context for the therapist as ethicist. The Reign of God, not modernity or postmodernity, is our liberating, culture-creating story. It provides the ethos and ethic for therapy and a critical, political perspective on Western culture.

- The church as a community can reflect the Reign of God in its practice and its conversation about what it means to be

Christian in the late twentieth century and into the next century. The church is not the Reign of God. But to the extent that the Christian community is significant, individualism and professionalism are made relative and appreciated.

- The individual is invited to reflect the Reign of God in personal character and in a life that is lived in wholeness in the Spirit. The therapist as ethicist is then called to be a person of character. And character is shaped by rituals, narratives, and the discernment of the Christian community.

Perhaps it is already apparent that a systems perspective is the framework that will shape the discussion of the relation of culture, religion, and psychotherapy. It is a perspective in the social sciences that has developed over the past several decades (Bateson, 1972, 1979; Hoffman, 1981; von Bertalanffy, 1968). A systems approach assumes that an individual or healer/psychotherapist is best understood in terms of ever-enlarging contexts or systems that range from the micro level to the macro level. Hence, one can move from an analysis at the biochemical level, to individual cognition, affect, and behavior, to family and neighborhood, to institutions, society, and international relations. It is assumed, in a systems perspective, that all systems are necessary for understanding the self, and that conflict between systems is inevitable, though harmony is the ideal.

A fundamental limitation of the systems approach is its rather pragmatic assumptions regarding ethics. If a system works, it is assumed that one best not tinker with it. However, as family therapists remind us, pathologically complementary families do "work." Thus, within each level of the system we need a normative analysis of what constitutes wholeness for culture, community, and the individual. I will examine the ethical dimensions of individual, community, and culture in relationship to a systems perspective on therapy, but the Reign of God will provide the ethical content for each of the three categories.

An Overview of the Journey

Allow me to sketch out in greater detail the three incarnational forms of the Reign of God. The first points to the crucial importance of God's presence in shaping a culture that promotes change. The second proposes that the church as Christ's body serves as an ethical context for therapy. The third focuses on the Spirit-driven character of the individual therapist as citizen of the Reign of God. There are, of course, other ways of interpreting the Reign of God (Snyder, 1991) but I will limit myself to these three in this book.

Culture

The individual therapist who seeks to be ethically sensitive is dependent on the moral ethos or resources provided by a culture. In both secular and religious psychological literature, there is almost complete silence regarding the public vision that shapes our practice. Generally we have focused on intrapsychic and interpersonal agendas rather than societal and cultural agendas. As a result one wonders how provincial our therapy and psychological anthropology really is. Is it possible, that unknown to us, primarily Western values determine the therapy we mediate?

The fundamental question shaping the first section of this book is "Therapy for what culture?" All therapy takes place in a cultural context. The therapist is shaped by culture and in turn reinforces it. Therapy is indeed a political process; that is, it is shaped by culture and it creates culture. Crucial, then, is a sense of the relation of the therapist to culture and a sense of how therapy differs with cultural context. Therapists would do well to examine carefully the cultural context of their thinking and practice and then commit themselves to the kind of culture they would consider normative. Would it really make a difference if therapy were shaped by a vision of the Reign of God as cultural? Can therapy help us discern when we need to be liberated from our culture or when to affirm it? To take the Reign of God seriously is to render all cultures relative.

Each chapter in Part 1 discusses the relationship of ethics to culture and therapy. The first chapter ("The Cultured Therapist") asks what ethical culture shapes the ethic of the individual therapist and his or her religious community. It asks how culture shapes the therapeutic process, and suggests that the form is ethical in nature. The biblical theme of the Reign of God will shape the discussion. This theme gives direction to the form, content, and process by which a religious ethos impacts healing and heal-

ers. The second chapter ("Psychology: The Gospel of Modernity?")
argues that cultures are ethical in nature and that the therapist
is an ethical agent of a particular culture. This chapter reflects
on the content of a particular culture—namely, North American
culture. The final chapter of this section moves from the form and
content of an ethical culture to one strategy by which an ethical
culture shapes therapy—namely, stories ("On Hearing and
Telling Stories").

Community

The individual therapist exists in a particular historical context. Until recently there has been an awkward silence about
the relationship of the therapist to his or her community. The
field of community psychology has raised our awareness of the
connection between therapy and community (Rappaport, 1977).
However, in religious circles we have assumed that physical
healing is so miraculous, and in secular settings that psychotherapy is so private, that the role of the community is
entirely secondary, if not irrelevant. These are dangerous
myths. Both therapist and therapy are inextricably connected
to communities. Both the therapist and the client are members
of some community whether they admit it or not. How do the
communities that the therapist accepts as normative shape the
healing process? What particular communities reinforce the
healing process?

As an ethicist, the religious therapist functions within ethical contexts that are communal in nature—the profession and
the religious community. The therapeutic process may well be
different, depending on whether the normative community that
serves as the primary context is the profession or the religious
community. The religious therapist who chooses the church
community may be in for a surprise, because if the church (as
the body of Christ) fails to discern and embody its convictions
and values, then the ethical language the Christian therapist
uses will have less clarity, meaning, or significance. If one
chooses the professional community as the primary ethical context of therapy, one may be shocked to discover that there is
little consensus on values, and that what is proffered is a minimalist ethic that shapes the form, not the content, of therapy.

The first chapter in Part 2 examines Western individualism as a critical obstacle to understanding the role of community in ethics and therapy ("That Individual"). The second chapter explores the role of the church as a community of ethical discernment and as a sign of the Reign of God ("Signposts along the Way"). The third chapter examines the ethical nature of professional communities ("Professional: To Be or Not to Be?"). Can one be authentically Christian and competently professional? The fourth chapter seeks to illustrate how the church can be a community of ethical discernment vis-à-vis the mental health profession ("A Community of Discernment"). It reviews five ways in which the church has historically related Christ to culture, and explores the implications for therapy.

Character

Part 3 focuses on the character of the healer. The character of the therapist and the process of therapy are connected. Perhaps the divorce of character from therapy and our obsession with technique is a consequence of a loss of soul and a loss of ethical vision.

The development of character is fundamentally dependent on the moral ethos of culture and the ethic incarnated by a specific community. If culture is fragmented and the community diffuse, the soul of the therapist may reflect this lack of center. This part of the book will ask in what way Western culture has shaped the character of contemporary healers. If the story of the Reign of God and the convictions of the Christian community are the normative context of the therapeutic process, what would be the character of the therapist?

Part 3 will focus directly on the personality of the counselor as a significant ethical context for therapy. It begins with a chapter on the nature of character ("On Character"). The chapter will focus directly on the nature of character as ethical personality. The second chapter examines the moral developmental theory of Lawrence Kohlberg, because it so quintessentially reflects the enlightenment paradigm and the modern ethos ("Enlightenment Morality Redux"). Then I will explore an approach I call pastoring our internal congregation as a way of developing character ("Pastoring Our Personal Congregations"). It is an attempt at a postmodern description of the pluralist self, filled with the substance of my faith heritage. The concluding chapter of the book provides the autobiographical basis of the ideas presented in Parts 1–3. Those who wish to begin with experience may wish to read it next ("Experiences between Jerusalem and Athens").

A Map for Whom?

In evangelical churches and the larger Protestant world, a distinction is made between lay caregiving, pastoral care, pastoral counseling, and Christian therapy. The differences among these roles tend to be based on setting, type of problems encountered, and level of expertise. Given the model proposed, all care that claims to be Christian is called to be consistent with the Reign of God, to reflect the convictions of the Christian community, and to embody in character the values of both. This is true whether a pastor is comforting a grieving family or a Christian psychologist is counseling a person with multiple personalities. To be sure, there is a difference in the experience and training of the therapist, but for both the direction is influenced by the degree to which their character is shaped by a vision of the Reign of God. There may be a difference in knowledge of symptomology, but each caregiver is part of an ethical community to which he or she is accountable. There may be variations in the length of training and availability of techniques, but the quality of the healer's character is still critical to the therapeutic process.

My Confessional Point of Departure

The model proposed here is written self-consciously, but not mechanically, from within a particular faith tradition. That tradition is variously referred to as the Believers' Church tradition (Durnbaugh, 1968), Baptist (McLendon, 1986), Free Church (Littell, 1952), or Anabaptist (Loewen, 1985). Denominations under the rubric of Believers' Church include Methodist, Brethren in Christ, Church of the Brethren, Mennonite, Plymouth Brethren, Disciples of Christ, Adventists, and Baptists.

The convictions of this array of churches first emerged as a response to the magisterial reformers of the sixteenth century. They shared with the Reformers a commitment to the

Scripture as an authoritative guide for the life of the believer. However, unlike the Reformers, they began with the call to discipleship as the center of the Christian life, rather than with Luther's emphasis on justification by faith. In contrast to the individualism of the Protestant reformers, the radical reformers focused on the body of Christ as a community of accountability. Entrance into the community of believers came not by infant baptism but by a voluntary confession of faith and a commitment to faithful obedience. Membership in the community of believers was represented not as a privileged status, but as a shared commitment to incarnate the ethic of Jesus.

The recognition of the plurality of the Christian world was a natural consequence of the persecution that followed when Anabaptists (i.e., rebaptizers) refused to baptize their infants. As a consequence, the Anabaptists called for a clear separation of church and state. I begin then with a respect for a theological and cultural pluralism that views the church and society as having many stories. Each story is told by individuals within particular communities with specific histories. The more particular our story, the more we recognize the particularity of all stories and the richer the dialogue between storytellers becomes.

My focus on ethics follows the impulse of the Believers' Church tradition, which tends to marry ethical injunction with theological reflection. James McLendon's definition of ethics is basic to the model presented in this book.

> Christians are a people formed by their shared convictions. As participants in a common story, they are bound together by convictions, moral convictions, about God and neighbor, about self and community, about where they have been and whither they are bound. Christian ethics must display the grammar of these convictions, or, to change the metaphor, must reveal the structure of the shared Christian story, if it is to offer critical insight about the moral life (1986:62).

However, to begin with ethics in a model for conversation between ethics and therapy does not mean that the focus will be on how to resolve ethical quandaries. Rather, as indicated above, I am more interested in the contexts that *enable* one to be ethical and that shape ethical convictions. Ethics here is concerned with community and culture as enabling contexts. My goal will not be to isolate the critical ethical principles that should shape practice; rather, I will focus on the narrative, the communal life, and personal rituals that help a therapist develop character consistent with the ethic of the Reign of God.

We could begin with principles such as the goodness of creation, the fallenness or goodness of human nature, the sanctity of human life, the equality of all persons, and so on. Such an emphasis on principles leads to a preoccupation with decisions made within the individual. It is this obsession with choice that Bonhoeffer (1954) suggested was a reflection of our fallenness, since it gives to the self the power of choice rather than seeing the self as an object of God's choice. My alternative is to begin with the cultural narratives, the communal conversations, and personal struggle for wholeness that are critical for healing to occur.

The model presented in this book is developed with the hope that theological ethics will be an articulate partner in our discussions of the nature of therapy. Because we have failed to take seriously the creation of alternative, explicit, and convincing religious and ethical frameworks, religious therapists have often unwittingly endorsed American culture as the primary universe of moral discourse. Clearly, we will not operate outside of the framework of Western culture, but perhaps we will be able to understand more clearly the ethic implicit in Western psychologies, and when there is continuity and when there is discontinuity. Ultimately, my hope is that the Reign of God will come on earth as it is in heaven.

Part 1

The Reign of God as an Ethical Culture

1

The Cultured Therapist

The opening speaker of the first "Evolution of Psychotherapy" conference hailed it as the "Woodstock of Psychotherapy." Some seven thousand therapists from twenty-nine countries gathered to listen to the experts in Phoenix in 1985, and again in Los Angeles in 1990. They were all there, from the outspoken family therapists such as Salvador Minuchin and Cloe Madanes, to the soft-spoken humanist-existentialists such as Viktor Frankl and Rollo May. The stylish hypnotherapists, Ernest Rossi and Jeffrey Zeig, were there. Object relations therapists were represented by James Materson, cognitive behaviorists by Donald Meichenbaum and Aaron Beck. And, of course, the gadflies were invited: Albert Ellis and Thomas Szasz. We saw them at their best (on video tape, of course) and at their worst (unloading their personal agendas on each other).

Beyond the variations indicted by their theoretical commitments, there were fundamental differences among them. Some were profoundly aware of the social context of the therapeutic process, others were not. Sophie Freud, granddaughter of Sigmund Freud, openly asserted that therapy is fundamentally a political process. She reminded us that therapists have tended generally to be blind to the effects of gender, race, and social status on the therapy process. Salvador Minuchin was concerned that some models of family therapy would not work with the poor. He should know, as he began his therapy with poor immigrant families. Minuchin presented a case to demonstrate the importance of the social context of therapy to the point where he advocated for a client in court (Elizur and Minuchin, 1989). Virginia Satir moderated an evening discussion on world peace at the 1985 conference. Thomas Szasz reminded the conferees that therapy in general, and these conferences in particular, were forms of socialization. These voices were, however, a minority. Most therapeutic approaches seemed unrelated to larger sociocultural considerations. Or, it was assumed the therapy of individual clients would in itself result in the creation of a more just and more therapeutic culture. Perhaps religiously oriented therapists assume this as well.

Being with a client in a rather small counseling room, it is possible to be entirely oblivious to the more invisible role of politics and culture. Politics is felt to be synonymous with senators, campaigns, and policy-making, not therapists, clinical interventions, and personal change. Therapy is generally assumed to be apolitical on the one hand, while touted as culturally sensitive and socially tolerant on the other.

One of the outstanding presentations at the second "Evolution of Psychotherapy" conference was that of James Hillman. The therapist and the client, he maintained, are citizens of national and international communities. He suggested that too often we remain political idiots even while we become more psychologically savant in therapy. For him therapy functions to dissolve provincialism. Therapy is always a communal, global, and cultural act. At present the therapeutic enterprise, in his view, is politically bankrupt (see Hillman and Ventura, 1992).

Implicit in every therapy is a vision of public morality—politics. Therapy communicates that vision by the metaphors it borrows, the symbols it uses, the stories it tells, and the rituals it prescribes. Implicit in that microcosmic event of therapy is a macrocosmic sociopolitical system. Therapy has political consequences. This position has been well stated by Halleck (1971). A therapist helps a patient find "the good life," not just in treating an emotional problem or simply enabling clients to cope with the environment. Halleck comments that "there is no way in which the psychiatrist can deal with behavior that is partly generated by a social system without either strengthening or altering that system. Every encounter with a psychiatrist, therefore, has political implications" (1971:36).

A major role of therapy in any culture is to reinforce the values of the culture. The "cultured" therapist is then one who affirms in his or her clients the deep structure of a given culture, its most profound values and ideas. Therapy is not simply helping people adjust to the surface demands of culture. The therapeutic enterprise is fundamentally cultural in nature.

Therapeutic Culture

A commonsense way of defining culture would be simply to talk about how one goes about living. It includes the rituals, traditions, and symbols that shape us (Frank, 1963; Luepnitz, 1988). Culture shapes the tone, character, and quality of our lives. It shapes our way of looking at the world that we consider common sense. It is factual, comprehensive, and, we hope, coherent. Culture provides a sense of personal identity. At its most powerful, culture is unconscious. Hence one might define culture as "a system of symbols which acts to establish powerful, pervasive and long-lasting moods and motivations in men by formulating conceptions of a general order of existence and clothing these conceptions with such an aura of factuality that the moods and motivations seem uniquely realistic" (Geertz, 1973:90).

The *curandero/curandera* is what one might call a "cultured" therapist in Mexican-American communities (Kiev, 1968). In this tradition therapy and illness are clearly experienced and understood within a particular cultural framework. While there are other diagnoses, a central diagnostic category has to do with the distress experienced in the process of acculturation to a North American culture. Therapy is clearly designed to reinforce traditional Mexican culture. Furthermore, the community of the healer plays a critical role in therapy. Not only are community members participants in the healing process; the goal of therapy is the return of the individual to this primary community. Also, Kiev points out, the charisma of the healer is a consequence of incarnating the religious beliefs and norms of the community. The character of the *curandero/curandera* is consistent with the ideals of the Mexican-American community. In fact, this tends to be the primary test of genuineness. The *curandero/curandera* is trusted by the community and given authority. He or she is an example of a cultured therapist.

It should come as no surprise, if an African-American therapist were being consulted, that the outcome of therapy might include an awareness of, appreciation of, and perhaps even commitment to African-American culture. Feminist therapists assume that consciousness raising about the roles of women and men in society is integral to the therapeutic process, and that one of the hoped for consequences is a more egalitarian culture.

Therapy then does not occur in a cultural vacuum. It both shapes and is shaped by culture. Culture defines the nature and possibility of healing. Years ago Perry London (1964) reminded us that culture can influence the definition of personal needs, value terms, procedures, language, setting, goals, and outcomes of therapy. However, the absence of a coherent or just culture undermines the therapeutic process. Fred Bloom, in the *Yale Review,* confesses that "in my own day-to-day attempt to provide a meaningful psychotherapy, I find myself increasingly thwarted by the reality outside the therapy, by the social and material culture of the patient and therapist, the ambiance, the setting, the milieu in which therapy takes place" (1977:3).

Culture as Morality

The existing resources in a given culture are the materials with which the culturally sensitive therapist labors, and which make therapy successful. The definition of culture given above by Geertz is actually not his definition of culture, but of religion. The fact that this definition seems to describe both religion and culture points to their fundamental similarity. Religion, like culture, can order a person's life through objective symbols and an articulated worldview, and it induces a distinct disposition. It seeks to help the individual at the points where chaos threatens to break in: to explain the inexplicable, to give meaning to suffering, and to provide moral insight.

Culture is not some interesting curio, the entertainment of vacations. We tend to treat culture as neutral, or as a matter of personal preference. Culture is then simply an entity created by anthropologists. However, the search for personal meaning is really a search for a meaningful culture to shape one's life. The potential contribution of culture to therapy is increased when culture provides a coherent universe of moral discourse, establishes a practical and just ethic, and trains the communal sensibilities of the individual to the point where they become habit. Rieff (1966) maintains that culture is fundamentally ethical and therapeutic in nature. Culture is the larger saving whole. A healthy culture provides for the individual (and for the therapeutic process) a relatively coherent worldview and a differentiated moral vocabulary. It does so by interpreting a particular activity in terms of some transcendent truth. A healing culture provides therapist and clients with a common center and common moral language.

Rieff (1966) maintains that at its best culture communicates ideas, makes distinctions between right and wrong, and provides a basic consensus. Traditional cultures created hedges for individual autonomy with a consensus of "shalt nots." There is, he suggests, a dialectic of "yes" and "no" that makes up the nature of culture. There is that which is affirmed/forgiven and that which is denied/rejected. Every culture creates its own balance of interdictions and remissions.

Following Freud, Rieff assumes that human nature is governed by instincts in need of control. He argues that civilization is built on coercion and renunciation. Thus culture at its best involves psychological retraining, an emptying of consciousness through asceticism. For this reason, Rieff referred to Freud as a moralist (1959). If it is successful, the antiinstinctual mode becomes pervasive and unconscious. Culture limits the spontaneous, establishes a level of adequacy of social functioning, and forestalls the danger of psychic collapse. Culture tames the wildness of experience by integrating the new into the old. The limitation of possibilities is the design of salvation.

A culture is therapeutic, Rieff argues, insofar as it provides remission (forgiveness) when communal purposes are violated. In a viable culture, whatever must be renounced disappears and is given back bettered. The process protects the individual against the panic and emptiness of normlessness. Rieff maintains that a viable culture is one that provides its members with mores that sink so deep they are commonplace. Providing reasons for behavior is then only the tip of the iceberg. It is historical institutions, not rational justifications, that create this interior understanding. At its best a culture/religion creates a sense of well-being, purpose, and freedom through affectionate and censorious authority.

A culture is therapeutic if it provides symbolic integration, a worldview, whether through art, science, religion, or philosophy. It is healing when it provides its healers with symbols in which the cultural superego is embodied. If a viable culture contributes to the healing process a coherent worldview and moral vocabulary, a concrete and compelling ethic, and a role model for the individual, then therapy cannot be viewed as a sanctioned retreat where culture/religion is irrelevant or to be excluded. Thus, with Rieff, I would say that if healing fails to occur one significant reason may well be that the cultural context either is not considered a resource, or that, in fact, it does not have resources to give.

Two Responses

Freud and Jung are two culturally sensitive therapists. Both assume that culture is a critical dimension of therapy. But there the similarities end. They have differing conceptions of the good society. They differ in regard to whether, or to what degree, the good society exists. They differ on the degree to which they believe existing culture *should* influence therapy. One finds Western culture oppressive, the other marvels at its moral resources resident in the individual. Freud and Jung are not alone among therapists in their views of culture. I will use them as representatives to illustrate these opposing perspectives of the role of culture in the therapeutic process.

First, there are those therapists who assume that culture is morally bankrupt and is, in fact, the cause of personal and social ills. Culture offers few, if any, resources for healing, emotional or moral. Its impact is moralistic. Therapy then has a strongly individualistic, heroic, or anticultural bias.

Freud was one of those with a pessimistic view of cultural resources for therapy. In his two later books *Civilization and its Discontents* (1936/1961) and *The Future of an Illusion* (1927/1961), he provides us with his interpretation of the relationship of ethics to culture. Positively, Freud argues that culture enables us to make the earth serviceable and protects us against the violent forces of nature. Culture provides order and thereby saves the individual from the necessity of having to make decisions. Culture attempts to regulate social relationships, rather than leaving them to the arbitrary will of the individual. It is able to do so because the community is stronger than the individual. However, because of a fundamental conflict between the needs of the individual and the demands of culture, the external world is, for Freud, threatening, cruel, and full of disappointments and impossible tasks. The goal of life is the happiness that comes from the alleviation of misery in our personal worlds. Happiness is the satisfaction of basic needs.

According to Freud, the most powerful technique devised by culture to control aggressiveness is the internalization of taboos-conscience. The superego directs aggressiveness toward the ego when external standards have been broken. The consequence is guilt and a desire to punish the self. The superego is simply an extension of external authorities. External authorities can only ask for the renunciation of instinct, while the superego creates guilt by equating the intention with the deed. Conscience is a product of instinctual renunciation by a loving authority who causes the standard to be internalized. Freud sought to represent the sense of guilt as the most important problem in the development of culture. The price we pay for our advance in culture is a loss of happiness through the heightening of the sense of guilt.

The psychoanalytic model begins with a positive view of the functions of culture but in the last analysis judges it as oppressive. The individual is in need of liberation from culture since social institutions are fundamentally coercive, particularly with regard to sexual mores. Religion, a potential resource, only serves the purposes of a controlling culture. Its function is to recompense the individual for deprivations experienced. The stance, then, toward culture as a healing resource is one of suspicion.

Freud assumed the necessity of order for culture to heal. As one might expect from one with Jewish roots, that order is not an abstract ethic; it is focused on the curbing of sexual desire and violent behavior. But still, the ethical demands of culture are too arbitrary and severe. Culture is potentially healing to the extent that it controls the individual, but in reality this control has been excessive. Culture has been oppressive, creating guilt-ridden individuals.

In contrast to Freud, there are those who find more healing resources in culture. It is assumed that there exists a moral consensus sufficient to support the therapeutic enterprise. There are clinicians who implicitly assume that Western culture is sufficiently endowed with moral resources to sustain the troubled individual. Unlike Freud, Jung (1933) assumes that Western culture has the ethical resources to heal and guide the troubled modern. To be sure, Jung was critical of its unquestioning faith in science, its shallow view of the human psyche, and its superficial view of evil. On the other hand, Jung's faith in the resources of the internal culture—i.e., the collective unconscious—stands in stark contrast to Freud's pessimism regarding the unresolved conflicts of culture residing in the unconscious.

For Jung, our lives are influenced by a reservoir of cultural resources (the collective unconscious). It is a repository of images and symbols that represent the human cultural heritage. Access to this repository comes through dreams and active imagination. Unlike Freud's individual, who is engaged in conflict and sacrifice for which recompense is sought, Jung's individual, particularly in the second half of life, is engaged in a significant search for meaning. The goal of this search is wholeness. Development is toward greater individuation and differentiation of the individual from the collective past.

Jung argues that the resources inherent in the collective unconscious are substantial and accessible to the individual. This cultural resource is a synthesis of the best in the history of culture. Jung is catholic in his use of Western and non-Western traditions. The healthy person is one with awareness of these cultural resources, who can contextualize his or her personal story in a larger cultural story. Jung assumes that the resources available to the self in the collective unconscious are, in fact, an ethical culture capable of guiding the modern soul. There is then a common ethical basis for conversation in the therapeutic hour. Jung does not regard the nature of ethical prescriptions as arbitrary, since they are not heteronomous but autonomous, not external but internal. Nor are they abstract,

since they are embodied in historical persons and cultural artifacts. The individual, for Jung, is not culture-free, but indeed,
is the carrier of culture. There is here no need to submit oneself to an objective, heteronomous external culture, but rather,
to the cultural resources within the self. Dreams and an analysis of their symbols provide the individual with the tools to
navigate modernity.

To summarize, for the "cultured" therapist, ethos and ethic
are inextricably linked. Cultured therapists make assumptions
about the nature of the good society, of culture. In turn culture
shapes the goals and provides the resources for therapy. A culture that heals needs a coherent moral vision and an organic
tradition. Early twentieth-century healers, such as Freud and
Jung, assumed a cultural coherence, but it was either too
oppressive or too liberating. The ethos of Western culture was
moralistic for Freud and compelling for Jung. However, both
assumed that the individual can and must transcend culture.

The Religious Context of Therapy

The "cultured" therapist, then, is one who understands that
culture is the context of therapy and that because culture is
essentially moral, therapy becomes *ipso facto* a moral enterprise. Before I examine the particular biblical theme of the
Reign of God as a cultural and sociopolitical context for therapy, I wish to explore more specifically culture as the moral
context to therapy. Bloom has lamented the loss of transcendence in psychotherapy. Transcendence, for him, involves the
"integration and reconciliation of the individual with a total
universe which is perceived to be alive with spiritual and moral
meaning. It is the resolution of a state of alienation with
respect to nature, mankind, the forces of creation, and the spiritual order of the cosmos" (1977:323).

In this regard the work of Don Browning (1976, 1983a,
1983b, 1988a, 1988b) deserves special attention. For almost
two decades Browning has lamented the loss of an ethical culture as the context of counseling—religious or secular. In his
seminal work, *The Moral Context of Pastoral Care,* he developed a model for pastoral care that I submit is applicable to
helping professionals in general. The thesis of his book is that a
pastoral care or therapy that presumes to be moral needs to be

understood within the context of a tradition of practical, moral rationality.

Browning turns to Judaism as a distinctively ethical type of religious culture to illustrate a tradition of moral rationality. Judaism approaches life with a type of practical rationality "that actively orders and seeks mastery over impulse and action in an effort to make them conform to the guidelines of certain practical rules of behavior" (1976:43). Browning argues that in Judaism human action is important in the transformation of culture. In the creation of an ideal society human action is capable of producing greater congruence between the ideal and the actual. Fundamental to Browning's approach is that therapy, like all acts of care, takes place in a moral, ethical context. Whether the acts of care are pastoral counseling or professional psychotherapy, whether secular or religious, there is a moral context that serves as a background. Secular therapists clearly assume a moral context in that there is a "more or less mutually recognizable and shared moral world that extends beyond the therapeutic situation and provides a moral horizon to the therapy, even though it may not be directly invoked by therapists in the process of counseling" (Browning, 1976:11). Too often, Browning laments, we have neglected the task of articulating and forming the larger moral universe. An ethical context makes a therapist's interventions interpretable. Failure to make this context explicit allows counselees to draw their own conclusions about the value context or to project their own idiosyncratic morality onto the therapist.

The myth of therapeutic neutrality and a fear of being judged moralistic have tended to make therapists play down the positive meaning frameworks of life and ethical resources that clients in fact bring to the counseling situation. Browning argues that when the moral frameworks of meaning about the various dimensions of life (such as interpersonal relations, death, illness, and aging) are clearer and explicit, the particular religious character of healing will also become clearer.

Browning has stated appropriately that acceptance, forgiveness, love, and community are meaningless and formless concepts without a context of moral norms, judgments, and structures. He makes the point that without a specific discussion of the nature of love, we are in a position of having community without structure. Hence, "we do not know whether love means giving another person a massage, sleeping with his wife, inviting him to a cocktail party, joining him for a potluck dinner, or what. We need to know the indices of love—the marks of love" (1976:79).

If there is no moral language functionally useful in the therapeutic context, then the focus of the conversation might well become exploration of inner trails as an end in itself. If therapists are blind to the fact that their therapeutic conversations occur in a moral/cultural context, they may well perceive their work as the application of amoral techniques. And if there are few ethical resources available culturally (MacIntyre, 1981), then the therapist and the therapeutic encounter must carry the freight of making the language of therapeutic dialogue morally practical and visible.

I could not agree more with Browning that healing requires a moral-ethical context to make it possible and intelligible. My model of the relationship of ethics to therapy tends to be less deontological and less abstract than that of Browning. Browning tends to focus on the wealth of practical laws that the Pharisees apply to everyday life. My approach is more confessional than systematic. It moves toward metaphors of story rather than moral rationality. Browning focuses on the practical moral rationality of Pharisaic Judaism, while I will take the story of the Reign of God as the central motif.

The Reign of God

Imagine a "cultured" therapist who wishes to take seriously Jesus' invitation to "seek first the Reign of God" (Matt. 6:33). Is culture, as I have defined it, incompatible with the biblical theme of the Reign of God? I shall contend that at one level there is continuity, but at another, possible discontinuity. The Reign of God has a cultural dimension, but it is not simply an extension of human culture. The foregoing plea for a moral context for therapy, for an analysis of the implicit ethical nature of culture, and for the recognition of the sociopolitical values that shape therapy lead me to take seriously the theme of the Reign of God as a response. I will assert that the Reign of God is a vision of an ethical culture that serves as a model for a society that can be a positive context for therapy.

To refer to the Reign of God as cultural and political context is to be more historically particular than to say in some general way that culture is the context of therapy. If the Reign of God is cultural and historical, it will take on the forms of tradition, ritual, symbol, worldview, ethos, and so on. In all these respects, however, the Reign of God is a culture both different from and similar to human culture. The theme of the Reign of God is to be in partnership with God in creating a people whose character reflects God's character. The biblical story is a story of God's creation of a unique people, a moral universe, a *specific culture*. The Reign of God is a story of God's breaking into history; it is, therefore, a political story. The Reign of God in the Old Testament is seen as a movement led by Yahweh. It is the announcement that God is coming (Ps. 18; Exod. 19). In the coming age, the rule of God will be universal (Isa. 52:10; Jer. 3:17), it will be righteous (Isa. 4:3-6; Jer. 31:31–34), and there will be peace (Isa. 2:2–4; 35:1–2).

The God of Abraham, Isaac, Rachel, and Esther is one who seeks to create a people. The Old Testament provides us with a description of ethical culture in general and with a preview of the structure of the Reign of God. The story begins with a promise to Abraham that his descendants shall be more numerous than the stars in heaven. The second major step in the creation of a people occurs with the exodus from Egypt. This people emerges out of slavery at the hand of Yahweh. The Sinai covenant marks the beginning of a special relationship between God and a people. Note that it is "a people" that is called, not simply individuals. Moreover, the people are called to become a *righteous* people whose character reflects the righteousness of their liberator.

The contribution of monotheistic religions is a monist view of culture, and the primary characteristic of monism is the demand for cultural coherence according to a central conviction. In the Old Testament that central conviction is that the transcendent God makes and keeps a covenant with a people. Ethical expectations that shape the character of the Israelite culture are made on the basis of the covenant that exists between Israel and Yahweh. Ethics begins with the hearing of a particular voice, not with some prior knowledge of what is right. In Old Testament ethics there is no prior, naturalistic definition of ethical terminology such as knowledge, justice, righteousness. The ethic is practical, not theoretical. It encompasses all of life.

God establishes a culture with a covenant that is both gracious and demanding. It invites humanity into a relationship in which they choose their ultimate loyalty and are invited to live their lives in such a way as to reflect this loyalty. The covenant made with humanity is one in which Yahweh promises faithfulness. There is here no rejection of law. A covenantal perspective will require that we reexamine the Old Testament story of God's people as the call to become a righteous people. An emphasis on peoplehood and law in the Old Testament does not mean that God is now distant, that law is simply guilt-producing, or that the Old Testament God accepts us conditionally. To understand culture as an ethical context of healing requires a recovery of the goodness of law (see Barth, 1959; Sanders, 1977).

The Reign of God depicted in the New Testament is an extension of the Old Testament vision for a righteous people of God. It is clearly political in nature. One needs only to read Mary's song (Luke 1:46–56). The Coming One will scatter the powerful and raise those of lowly status. Similarly, when Jesus returns to Nazareth he reads this text in the Synagogue:

> The Spirit of the Lord is upon me,
> because he has anointed me to preach the gospel to the poor;
> he has sent me to heal the brokenhearted,
> to preach deliverance to the captives,
> and recovery of sight to the blind,
> to set at liberty those that are bruised (Luke 4:18).

In so doing, Jesus sets forth a political program so offensive it leads ultimately to his death (Yoder, 1972). Proclaiming the Reign of God is the center of Jesus' purpose: "I must preach the kingdom of God to the other cities also, for I was sent for this purpose" (Luke 4:43). And it is what the disciples are mandated to proclaim (Luke 9:1–2). Baptism for Jesus was joining a movement, a new society guided by God (Luke 3:21–23). It was not enough simply to be a Jew. It symbolized consistency with the purposes of God in the world.

The primary mission of Jesus was to gather God's endtime people to be the Church. Jews—and Jesus was no exception—

thought in terms of nations and peoples. The image is that of exiles returning to Jerusalem with God leading them (Isa. 52). Thus Jesus chose twelve disciples to symbolize the twelve tribes of Israel. He healed people—the restoration of God's people. Jesus taught people to pray, which is the mark of God's people. The Reign of God is to be a concrete, historical reality. It is rooted in history; hence, the political contexts of Jesus' birth are given (Luke 2:1–3; 3:1). But the Reign of God is also future, to be fulfilled. There is always a tension between the ideal and the real. This tension precludes an accommodation to the present age. The Reign of God is historical but also symbolic: present and not present.

While the Reign of God is the creation of a particular culture, it is also universal. Jesus is the redeemer of the whole world and thus Luke traces his genealogy to Adam (3:1–2, 6, 38). Membership in the Reign of God is composed of all people (Luke 2:10), Samaritans (Luke 9:51–56; 10:30–37; 17:11–19), pagans (Luke 2:32; 3:6, 38; 4:25–27; 10:1, 24–47), Jews (Luke 1:33; 2:10), Gentiles (Luke 4:25–27; 13:29; 24:47), publicans and sinners (Luke 3:12; 5:27–32; 7:37–50; 19:2–10, 23, 43), respectable people (Luke 7:36; 11:37; 14:1), the poor (Luke 1:53; 2:7; 6:20; 7:22), the rich (Luke 29:2; 23:50), women and men (Luke 10:38–42).

Jesus' vision of an alternative culture emerges in the context of other political visions for an oppressed people available in his own day (Yoder, 1972). The Pharisees' program was the creation of a holy people separated by a regimented program of disciplines. The Sadducees collaborated with the Romans to maintain the status quo in Palestine. The Zealots, at the other extreme, sought the overthrow of the Romans through violence. The Essenes proposed another option, that of complete isolation. Jesus rejected each of these political options for the renewal of Jewish culture. It was the Pharisaic option that Jesus interacted with most often and clearly rejected (Borg, 1984). In contrast to Browning's suggestion that the ethic of the Pharisees became a model for the healing process, I would suggest that, while the Pharisees understood the importance of ethics and culture, it was a combination different from that of Jesus' view of the Reign of God. Both sought the renewal of Judaism, but the content and process of its re-creation were different.

To make clearer the social and political nature of the Reign of God, I will contrast the platform of the Pharisees and Jesus (Borg, 1984). The dominant way of creating distinctive identity for the Pharisees in the face of Roman occupation was an emphasis on holiness. So the Pharisees focused on Torah and Temple. Holiness meant separation, hence the obsession with Sabbath observance, tithing, and ritual purity. That was the only road to the survival of Jewish culture, the Pharisees insisted, in an overpowering Roman culture. Only then would Israel be insulated from the corrosive influence of Romanism.

Like the Pharisees, Jesus was concerned about the purpose of the people of God in culture, their collective historical life. In contrast, Jesus represents a gentler, more inclusive program for a righteous and just culture. The fact that Jesus had a different political program resulted in a clash over differing visions of what the people of God should look like. That he was a threat to the other renewal movements is obvious from the events that led to his death.

The contrast between Jesus and the Pharisees is not simply between genuine and false personal piety. Jesus' conflict with the Pharisees was due to competing ethical visions of Israel's future, not simply their offensive legalism. The conflict was most evident over observance of holiness codes regarding table fellowship, the sabbath, and the temple. To eat with someone was to be intimate. For the Pharisees the meal must be pure. One could not eat with someone who had not tithed, or partake of food that had not been consecrated. Table fellowship was thus a symbol of what Israel would be among the nations: separate and holy. For example, Jesus' eating with tax collectors, prostitutes, and sinners created incredible opposition.

Jesus' relationship with specific persons also created conflict for the Pharisees because it represented a different political paradigm, a different vision of renewed Jewish culture. Sinners, for Pharisees, were those people of certain occupations (seven, to be exact!), who were immoral, who violated the Pharisees' commandments, as well as those who were Gentiles. A renewed Jewish culture would be exclusive. Jesus responded by saying that the sick, not the well, need a doctor. The lost (e.g., Zacchaeus) needed to be restored into the community. Jesus invited the rejected to celebrate with him (Luke 15).

Jesus' new society was the development of a new, more inclusive culture.

Thus, the tension between exclusion and inclusion became a key plank in Jesus' political platform. The cultured Pharisees had extended the holiness code for priests to all people. Thus when Jesus and the disciples ate food with unwashed hands, they objected. Jesus said that nothing from the outside that enters defiles; but only what is inside. Thus Jesus denied the foundation of the Pharisees' political program of separation and holiness. The Pharisees were busy paying tithes (Luke 11:42), but they were unconcerned about justice, mercy, and faithfulness (Matt. 23:23). They neglected the love of God. In the story of the Good Samaritan (Luke 10), it was the fear of defilement that kept the priest and Levite from helping. The prayer of the Pharisees (Luke 18:10ff) is not simply self-righteousness. Jesus' affirmation of the tax collector's prayer was a rejection of the Pharisees' program of separation (fasting and tithing). Jesus calls them leaven (Luke 12:1), unmarked graves (Luke 11:44), blind guides (Luke 6:39), and those who simply preserve the truth but are unproductive (Luke 19:12–27). They immersed themselves in the Torah but forgot that it was *life* that the Reign of God would bring (John 5:39).

Jesus' program for cultural renewal was that of mercy, justice, and faithfulness to God. The theme of mercy rather than holiness appears in the prayer of the tax collector, in the story of the Good Samaritan, and in the Prodigal's father. Jesus quotes Hosea 6:6, "I prefer mercy, not sacrifice," and states "Be merciful even as your father is merciful" (Matt. 5:38–48) in parallel to "Be holy as your father is holy" (Lev. 19:2). Mercy is *hesed,* a covenant word. It points to the fact that God established and sustains a covenant with humanity to create a unique people. It is inclusive in that God makes rain to fall on the just and the unjust.

The Pharisees assumed that God's mercy was limited to the Hebrew people. For Jesus, mercy was to be applied in their historical situation—to the Romans. In Leviticus (19:18), love of neighbor meant love of fellow Israelites, but for Jesus it meant love of the non-Jew, even one's personal enemy. Thus Jesus says to go the second mile if compelled to go one mile by a Roman soldier. Jesus' ethic is specific not abstract. Those who show mercy will be "called the sons of God" (Matt. 5:45). Even the Gentiles love those who love them. Thus the program of Jesus is not resistance to the Romans, but inclusion. Borg (1984) argues that with Jesus there is a shift in the meaning of *hesed*. Where previously it meant steadfast loyalty within a covenant, now it meant inclusiveness.

So then, the "cultured" therapist who seeks first the Reign of God is one who knows that the biblical story of the Reign of God is about culture. But the Reign of God is not any ordinary culture. It may well conflict and argue with other conceptions of the good society. "To seek first the Reign of God" for the "cultured" therapist means that the vision, story, events, and characters of the Reign of God are the normative context, the primary story for understanding the nature of therapy. This is a culture that is characterized by mercy, justice, and faithfulness to God. Jesus assumes that healing and the inbreaking of the Reign of God are related. When the Reign of heaven comes in its fullness, it will be like a small mustard seed that becomes a large tree (like a culture) and its branches a place to rest (therapeutic).

He told them another parable:

> The kingdom of heaven is like a mustard seed, which a
> man took and planted in his field.
> Though it is the smallest of all your
> seeds, yet when it grows, it is the largest of
> garden plants and becomes a tree, so that the
> birds of the air come and perch in its branches (Matt. 13:31–32).

Some Contemporary Voices

In the history of the church, a chorus of voices have called for a Christian culture. They have understood that the form of the Reign of God is that of an ethical culture. Its morality is practical and shapes everyday life. These individuals understand that in the Old Testament God's covenant was not simply with an individual but with a people, and that ultimately all the nations of the world are to be blessed by Yahweh. They know that Old Testament law, the Wisdom literature, the Sermon on the Mount, and Paul's exhortations to the Mediterranean churches are intended to give body to the ethic of the Reign of God.

A vision for the reign of God *on earth* has many proponents. Augustine's vision was the establishment of the city of God on earth. His writings became the floor plan for Constantinian and Medieval Christianity. For centuries Catholicism created a common religion that stretched across continents and nations. John Calvin held to this view of Christianity by establishing a theocracy in Geneva.

T. S. Eliot had a clear sense of the Reign of God as ethical culture. In his classic essay "The Idea of a Christian Society," Eliot (1940) suggests the outlines of such a culture. It is a society, not of saints, but of ordinary people whose Christianity is communal before being individual. For Eliot a Christian society is one in which every dimension of life has been touched by a central vision.

Similarly, Nicholas Wolterstorff (1983) has called for a "world-formative Christianity." It is his hope that the individual Christian will see his or her work in relationship to the creation of Christian culture. He states,

> The saints are responsible for the structure of the social world in which they find themselves. That structure is not simply part of the order of nature; to the contrary, it is the result of human decision, and by concerted effort it can be altered. Indeed, it should be altered, for it is a fallen structure in need of reform. The responsibility of the saints to struggle for reform of the social order in which they find themselves is one facet of the discipleship to which their Lord Jesus Christ has called them, it is not an addition to their religion; it is there among the very notions of Christian spirituality (1983:3).

In Wolterstorff's view, Christians are called to struggle to establish a holy commonwealth here on earth.

Parker Palmer (1988) in his book *The Company of Strangers* invites Christians to take seriously their responsibility for public life. Public life is what I have referred to as culture and sociopolitical structures. Public life is the life we have in common with strangers, with individuals who may never recognize God as creator and redeemer but who nonetheless are made in God's image. It includes the people of the earth whose common lot we share. The public (read culture) is a result of labor invested in the other without self-interest. It is what results when we interact with a wide range of people in our neighborhoods or in work settings, whether with the Red Cross, at the county fair, or in open debate. The public is what we have in common with all others. Here is the setting where mutual aid becomes possible, where people are drawn out of themselves. Society is the context where our ideas are expressed and tested. The public is where our projects are attempted.

So What?

This chapter began with the lament that psychologists, whether secular or religious, too often suffer from cultural myopia. I proceeded then to make a case for the "cultured" therapist as one who is politically aware, socially responsible, and culturally sensitive. I have asserted that for the therapist who wishes to take seriously the mandate to "seek first the Reign of God," it means understanding the Reign of God in a cultural sense, not only in a personal sense. Too often religion is doled out in bits and pieces. Religion is no seamless cloth blanketing the life of the religious or not-so-religious person's life. I have suggested that the Reign of God can be envisioned as that blanket—as a culture. What are the implications for therapy?

1. To emphasize the cultural context of healing and the biblical theme of the Reign of God is to say that therapy requires more than focusing on *internal processes.* Culture is a program for how to live—ethics. An ethical context for psychotherapy will involve not only an articulation by the therapist and his or her community of the nature of love, forgiveness, and grace; but also engaging ethical discernment, developing a common moral vision, and accepting accountability to others. A context that is perceived as both ethical and cultural/political will enable therapists to see pathology in a cultural and ethical perspective.

Because religion degenerates so easily into moralism, and perhaps because of a disenchantment with their moralistic religious upbringing, many therapists (whether evangelical or liberal) have rejected the ethical dimension of their faith heritage and have retained the internal, more emotive, and accepting dimensions. In the absence of a coherent, moral-ethical ethos and an acceptable process of moral discernment that truly shapes everyday life, the therapist easily focuses more on internal processes than on public responsibility, and consequently therapy may take on an antinomian, anticultural character.

2. To emphasize the cultural dimension of therapy and the Reign of God points to a *public responsibility*. Politics addresses the plight of the poor, the disenfranchised, the neglected. Yet, for those who are clinicians, work occurs almost exclusively in a private setting. The public, presumably, does not directly intrude. Even granted the importance of confidentiality for the sake of the client, we are still faced with the problem of public accountability for what transpires in private. We can lose our sense of connectedness to the larger social whole. The point of this chapter is that as "cultured" psychologists we are called to a public responsibility, and that the content of this public response can be shaped by the biblical vision of the Reign of God. This requires a translation of religious language into the language of the public. One task of the psychologist as Christian is the development of a public vision driven by Christian convictions.

3. The political agenda of the Reign of God as an ethical culture is indeed *relevant* to our culture and in turn to the therapeutic process. Specifically, I refer to issues of gender, wealth, and power (Foster, 1978, 1985). If the Reign of God is the goal of therapy, then any therapeutic approach that is repressive of women is unacceptable. A therapist who perpetuates power relationships through manipulative techniques is unethical. A mental health system that provides assistance only to the wealthy perpetuates the ideology that wealth is power. This too is unsatisfactory. To say that the Reign of God is the implicit goal of therapy has implications for the direction of therapy.

4. Another implication of articulating a connection between the cultural context for therapy and the Reign of God is once again to critique the myth of *neutrality* in therapy. To accept the Reign of God as context implies that the assumptions and procedures of the healing process in the larger cultural context are not neutral. The American cultural context in which we function is also an ethical culture. Too often religious psychologists and pastoral counselors have blissfully ignored this cultural context; they have too often focused on bringing psychological insights to a provincial church. We forget that the culture of a "People of God" is not synonymous with North American culture.

All therapy is a process of socialization into a culture. The question then is, "which culture?" The therapist who begins with the confession that the Reign of God is his or her primary context for therapy implies that the direction of therapeutic process will be influenced in a gentle way by that commitment. No, this does not mean that the values are automatically imposed upon the client. It does mean that the therapist is aware of his or her larger ethical commitments. It means these commitments are consistent with the biblical story of the Reign of God.

One might ask Jung whether the culture he trusts is a just culture. What Jung did not do is critique Western culture from a perspective beyond itself. To use the past to provide the ego with identity requires at least that we ask which mythic past is worth identifying with, which symbols are normative, viable, good, or appropriate. It is not clear whether a vision of a good society shaped how Jung selected myths to interpret archetypes. To choose history as the source of normativity raises the possibility of reinforcing the *status quo*. A clear vision of the "Reign of God" as a culture can be a corrective.

5. When the cultural context of therapy is explicit and the culture is relatively more coherent, just, and valued by both therapist and client, the therapist need not make direct reference to it. It does its work *quietly*. The client and the therapist have a common reference point, a common moral language, common ideals. However, what if the therapist has a point of departure different from that of the dominant culture or the client's culture? I believe that the therapist who "seeks first the Reign of God" has a fundamental responsibility to assist in the process of creating a public moral-ethical context so that his or her interventions are also interpretable within that framework. Failure to make this context explicit allows counselees to draw their own conclusions about the content of our therapeutic language or to project their own idiosyncratic morality onto it. To begin with the Reign of God as the context of therapy is to create a climate where the deepest spiritual yearnings of a client can be expressed.

6. The Reign of God context gives substantive *meaning* to the ethical terms that emerge in the therapy. Our contemporary therapeutic vocabulary includes such ethically laden terms as the following: self-actualization, wholeness, being

human authenticity, congruence, self-acceptance, guilt, good communication, differentiation, freedom, enmeshment, and growth. Note how abstract these terms are. They do not declare their ethical content. As a result of the absence of a culturally embodied moral language, and the cultural dominance of emotivism, we have no rational way of filling our moral language with content. Too often modern therapists nonetheless remain confident that the substance of their moral expressions is understood (e.g., to love, to accept, to tolerate, etc.). And when ethical commitments are merely personal preferences, building a common moral language with a client is a difficult, if not impossible, process. It is assumed that either the client or the therapist will fill, or is capable of filling, ethical terms with ethical content.

Browning (1976) has appropriately observed that acceptance, forgiveness, love, and community are meaningless and formless concepts without a cultural and moral context of norms, judgments, and structures. The moral content of our ethical terms can take their meaning from the culture in which they are used and/or from the content of the story of God's people. However, our moral vocabulary will remain abstract unless we take seriously the way ethical language is incarnated in Christ's life and in the life of the church. When there is embodiment, the Christian therapist can use the language with integrity and with effect.

Does that mean we use only the language of faith in therapy? No. Clients bring their moral vocabulary (as do therapists), and the meaning of these terms is derived from the culture in which they live. We begin with where a client is, but we do not end there. Every therapist as therapist makes an addition. For example, when the writer of the book of John (1:1–11) uses the language of *logos,* he fills it with new meaning: no longer is logos simply the rational principle that governs the universe; the rational principle becomes here the incarnate Son of God. Similarly, the therapist who seeks first the Reign of God begins with the moral language of the client but is aware of more meanings, and cocreates new meanings with the client.

The way in which the additional meanings shape therapy is complex. One can translate and use the categories in such a way that a listener understands. For example, one can fill the ethical term "assertiveness" with additional content (self-confidence AND self-sacrifice). Such a process is inevitable when one crosses cultures from Jerusalem to Athens. To move from the story of the Reign of God to modernity or postmodernity is such a cultural shift. Like the *curandero/curandera,* the feminist, or any culturally sensitive therapist, one listens to the language of one's counselees from the perspectives of the client caught in one culture and yearning for a different one. Once the ethic of the Reign of God is a given, one is free to work at a variety of ways that, without imposition, will make available to a client the healing culture of the Reign of God.

7. But, to be realistic, is the vision of the Reign of God as a culture one that can shape the therapeutic process in the modern world, given the powerful influence of existing cultures? If there are no communities that in a preliminary way incarnate the values of the Reign of God, then the influence of prevailing culture will dominate. Where the values of the existing culture are congruent with the "Reign of God," then we can gratefully accept them. However, where there is a conflict between the existing culture and the values of the Reign of God, more is required than simply asserting a different value. What is required is cultural and historical *embodiment.*

2

Psychology: The Gospel of Modernity?

While directing a study program in Mexico some years ago, I visited the national university in Mexico City. I was awed with its imposing architecture, size (200,000 students), and advanced psychology department. While browsing in the bookstore, I noticed that psychology books consumed more than a quarter of the space for student texts. I was intrigued. Why such interest in psychology? I began examining the textbooks. It appeared that most of the books used in the university were translations of American textbooks. Some introductory texts were written by Mexicans, but they reviewed primarily research with subjects who lived in the United States. There were very few books written by Mexican authors about research studies with Mexican subjects. A small number of authors attempted to develop an indigenous psychology. One might well conclude that one of the factors that will shape an emerging Mexican consciousness will be an awareness of American psychology and its worldview. If Western psychology reflects Western ideals, then it should come as no surprise that Western psychology will assist, for better or for worse, in the process of socializing emerging nations into modernity. However, as I have argued in the last chapter, culture is not neutral, it is ethical in sum and substance. In the past century Western Christian missionaries were accused of being the carriers of Western culture. Now the missionaries are McDonalds, sitcoms, and modern Western psychology!

I have suggested in the previous chapter that there is an existing cultural (i.e., ethical) context to psychotherapy and that the biblical story of the Reign of God speaks to that context. I suggested that a commitment to making the Reign of God a priority has clear implications for the way one interprets the discipline of psychology and the practice of psychotherapy. If indeed the Reign of God finds cultural and political expression and the field of psychotherapy is also ethical and cultural, then one might expect an interesting conversation between the two. This chapter intends to engage in that dialogue. If Christianity and psychotherapy are viewed apolitically then this conversation is unnecessary. I assume that both are culturally influenced and that dialogue is necessary. There are dimensions of modern American culture that are consistent with the themes of the Reign of God, and there are dimensions that are inconsistent.

The conversation is not unlike persons from different cultures comparing and contrasting experiences and customs. If the individuals conversing assume that their respective cultures are really identical, then obviously the contribution of one to the other is minimized. It wouldn't be the first time faith commitments and a specific culture have been confused in the history of Christianity.

I would like to make the case that psychology and Christianity in North America reflect in varying degrees modern culture. Both need the *qualifying* perspective of the Reign of God described in the previous chapter. We cannot engage in meaningful dialogue between faith and discipline unless we are willing to admit the cultural limitations (if not encapsulation) of the discipline of psychology and our interpretations of truth. The dialogue, to be fruitful, demands humility on the part of both partners since both are shaped by a particular (if not provincial) ethic/culture.

North American culture becomes the normative context of therapy and faith when there is no alternative context to therapy. The biblical theme of the Reign of God provides that alternative for those who seek it first. It enables us to affirm those elements of culture and religion that are consistent with or an extension of the ethic of the Reign of God. I do, however, begin with the assumption that there will always be some tension between the ethic of the Reign of God and the cultures that organize our experience. When there is no tension, we have capitulated.

In the previous chapter we focused on the cultural context of therapy. An individual is shaped by culture and also shapes culture. Thus health care professionals and institutions influence the ethos of a culture and are shaped by that ethos. This is the case whether they are religious or secular, whether they are scholars or therapists. In this chapter we concentrate on how culture shapes knowledge and practice. Knowledge and practice, whether psychological or theological, do not emerge out of a vacuum. No therapy, secular or religious, remains uninfluenced by the stories culture provides. If it is the case that all individuals are significantly shaped by their cultural background, why should that be any different if the individual is a psychologist or social worker, a Christian therapist or pastoral counselor?

To illustrate in a general way how the American psychologist and psychological knowledge are bound by the North American cultural story we can examine how psychologists function cross-culturally. Conflict may emerge when the story or vision of the ideal society in the host country clashes with the one contained in the imported North American psychology. Zuniga (1975) has described the inability of psychologists trained in the U.S. to assist in the social development of Chile during the turbulent 1970s. The psychologists were unable to cope with the politicization of their research or to provide an adequate rationale for their social projects or commitments. Their research modalities often clashed with the assumptions of larger national agendas. Often psychologists simply assumed modernization along Western lines. They were unaware of the politically charged assumptions that guided the definition of a problem, the methods of studying the problem, the interpretation of data, and the utilization of results. Zuniga concludes, "the ethnocentrism in the training of American psychologists which is ever-present but irrelevant for all practical purposes suffers a radical transformation when it is mechanically transported to a different cultural context. What was only a localized deficiency becomes a universalistic ideology and an unconscious (or guilt-ridden) advocacy of a cultural intrusion that is often extremely naive" (1975:105). Zuniga adds that psychologists were the least politically aware of the Western social scientists coming to his country.

A similar point has been made so often of Western missionaries that the litany of complaints need not be repeated. It should not be assumed that the Christian community is the innocent partner in the dialogue with psychology and that only the psychologists reflect the "world." Our age is not the first in which the church has been willing to sacrifice its identity for the sake of other gods. When the church is primarily concerned about its own survival it may well lose its identity entirely by succumbing to modernity. The church has too often been concerned about oiling the machinery of its own institutions rather than carefully asking what it means to be the church in the twentieth century. Failure to reflect on the church's identity in the context of culture will only result in indiscriminate borrowing that in the end will undermine the life and vision of the church community (Ellul, 1967).

Western theologians have also been criticized for their lack of awareness of the provinciality of their theology. Third world theologian, Miguez-Bonino (1975), has urged first world theologians to recognize their ideological bias. If the story line of American psychology and Christianity socializes people in other cultures, one wonders what impact American psychology and Christianity has had on its native soil. Have they served as socialization agents for those who are learning to walk in step with modernity? Science, technology, capitalism, pluralism, and individualism are some of the more obvious dimensions of modernity. Psychology as a discipline and Christianity as a social entity are influenced by these dimensions of modernity and reinforce them. The Canadian psychologist Lewis Brandt (1970) and the American psychologist Edward Sampson (1977) are probably correct when they argue that the science of psychology is largely a result of the American way of life. The question we can then ask is in what ways are psychology and psychotherapy a reflection of a particular culture—modernity.

Some Reflections on Culture and Knowledge

Before I proceed to an analysis of the relationship of psychology to the Western social/ethical context, some reflections on the relationship of knowledge to society are in order. Knowledge, psychological or theological, is influenced by a specific historical context (Gurvitsch, 1971; Habermas, 1972; Jacoby, 1975). Its nature reflects in varying degrees the ethos of a particular culture. Knowledge not only emerges out of a specific historical and social context, it also shapes and reinforces the worldview of that culture. The effects of society and knowledge are thus reciprocal (Mannheim, 1936; Berger and Luckman, 1966). The relationship between knowledge and society is therefore complex. In order to disentangle the process and effects of knowledge creation, one must examine a number of factors. First, there are a variety of social contexts that influence knowledge construction. Most broadly, there is the cultural ethos. Psychology as a scientific discipline, for example, has emerged in the past hundred years in primarily Western, industrialized countries. Theology as a discipline has been dominated by male writers. Then there are the more specific contexts of social position, class, generation, occupational role, ethnic affiliation, or group structures (e.g., university, seminary, sect, political party). From this perspective, psychologists and theologians are usually middle-upper class, urban, professional, male, and Caucasian. The predominant context has been the university setting, though since World War II psychologists have moved more into the areas of government and business, and over the years theologians have moved to seminaries.

The academic community is an example of one of these more specific social contexts. Thomas Kuhn (1970) expanded the argument that knowledge is a function of one's professional community. These communities, he maintained, are integrated by paradigms that have an internal coherence and that shape the questions, methods, and content of scientific inquiry. Kuhn refers to the shift from one paradigm to another as a revolution. Members of the community become committed to a particular set of beliefs that are difficult to lay aside until the evidence is so overwhelming that the prevailing paradigm is no longer adequate. Such a community of scholars has developed a common way of looking at the world as a consequence of their professional training, their common methodology, their consensus on critical problems, and their agreement on primary values. Such a community and the knowledge it creates seeks to be legitimated in the society in which it happens to exist. It also seeks to make a contribution to it.

In both the psychological and theological communities there are smaller universes of meaning that serve to shape the selection of admissible knowledge: cognitive psychology, process theology, object-relations theory, cognitive dissonance theory, narrative studies, behaviorism, Christology, scientific psychology, exegetical studies, critical psychology, or liberation theology. Psychologists function within a given universe of discourse. So do theologians. In the last century theology has been nurtured in the university and seminary settings. How has that setting shaped its reflections? To the extent that these institutions reflect Western culture and are isolated from some populations (the poor or women), it should not come as a surprise that theology is shaped by culture.

Psychologists and theologians, psychotherapists and pastoral counselors, have been slow to recognize the particularity, the cultural limitations, of their knowledge. It would appear that they have not been very self-conscious about the way society shapes the nature of knowledge and in turn how knowledge influences the shape of society. Thus the study of the social contexts of psychological knowledge (a new enterprise in itself) is only the beginning. In a seminal paper entitled "The Emerging Field of a Sociology of Psychological Knowledge," Buss (1975) has made the case that "we need to begin understanding the role of politics, ideologies, values, economic systems, and in general, society and its underlying structure and dynamics—in the birth, development, and death of some classic psychological theories, perspectives, paradigms, models, or approaches that have or continue to exert considerable influence" (1975:991). Both the discipline and practice of psychologists and theologians exist in particular social contexts. They occupy a particular social position, are members of a variety of organizations, and play a variety of socially prescribed and sanctioned roles. As individuals who have been educated in Western schools, they are socialized in varying degrees into particular cultural perspectives. The consequence is that they possess a knowledge base that reflects in part the structure of their social existence—modernity. The ahistorical perspective of much of current theological and psychological inquiry seems to be a result of our attempt to imitate the natural sciences and a desire to transcend the particular. Yet unlike natural scientists, psychologists deal with facts that are largely nonrepeatable and that fluctuate markedly over time. Theologians deal with concepts that are empirically nonverifiable. The principles of human interaction cannot be readily developed over time because the context within which they occur does not generally remain static.

Based on the above discussion I conclude the following: psychological and theological constructs are not unrelated to historical processes of modernity. Consequently, to characterize psychological and theological knowledge in idealist, ahistorical terms is less helpful. However, knowledge cannot be simply reduced to social or economic processes. There is a dialectical relationship between ideas and culture. Further, if knowledge is intimately related to culture, then the relationship to the Reign of God as an alternative cultural vision deserves serious attention.

The Premodern and Modern Cultural Contexts

The broader story that shapes both Western psychologies and theologies is the shift from traditional to modern existence. This story begins in the distant past when we were "traditional," and moves to the present where we are "modern." I am quite aware that there is considerable discussion about the emergence of a postmodern culture and that an analysis of Christianity and psychology in terms of modernity may be obsolete. I will not examine postmodernism in this chapter for several reasons. The most important reason is that most of Western psychology and theology is still largely a reflection of modernity. Second, if we understand the connection between modernity and knowledge, the reader will be able to apply the same approach to postmodernism and the disciplines of psychology and theology. I assume that an analysis of psychology in terms of modernity is prior and that reflections on postmodernity are still needed.

Toennies (1957) describes two forms of social existence: *Gemeinschaft* (community) and *Gesellschaft* (society). These two forms correspond to traditional and modern societies. Premodern societies, the narrative tells us, are rooted in agriculture and close to the natural world. In varying degrees, they possess common beliefs, rituals, and traditions. Continuing membership comes by conformity. Kinship ties are strong, village life is central, and mutual aid is common. Order is maintained by folkways and mores, while knowledge tends to emerge from religion and experience. The family is the economic unity and primary basis for socialization of its members into the values of the culture. The individual in this community is secure but not highly differentiated. The survival of the community supersedes the individual's needs.

The modern world is a new development in the story. It is no longer the land, but machines that are now the focus. Not the cultivation of soil, but the transformation of nature is the goal. Accumulation of wealth becomes more abstract. Diversity in belief, custom, and tradition is celebrated. Kinship ties are replaced with professional connections and block parties. Order is maintained by law based on contract. Knowledge is grounded now in observation, universal laws, and the awareness of common symbols. The school and peers play a greater role in the socialization of children. Abstract rationality is prized over intuition and common sense. The individual is the primary unit, economically, ethically, psychologically, and politically. Society, then, is the aggregate of enlightened individuals in the pursuit of happiness. For professionals, the profession replaces the ethnic group as the primary community. Central to an understanding of modernity is its loosening of social bonds. Relationships between people are regulated more by contracts than covenants. Religion, work, freedom, and equality are interpreted from an individual perspective. It becomes virtually impossible in the modern world to develop communities with a set of common beliefs, rituals, and traditions. Residual social structures are experienced as moralistic and repressive.

If one reflects on contemporary psychology and Christianity in relation to this grand plot, one can better understand the nature of the dialogue between them. While this plot is much more intricate than described here, it is nonetheless the case that this shift is repeated in history and recapitulated in our day with each wave of immigrants. The process of urbanization in many ways mirrors this movement from *Gemeinschaft* to *Gesellschaft*. It is obvious in the socialization of ethnic groups into Western culture. I do not, however, assume that the shift from premodernism to modernity is universal or an invariant process in all cultures.

Modernity, Psychology, and Theology

In a general way psychology reflects the story of the West. American society reflects the modern ethos and modernity is the primary context of contemporary psychology and theology. It is hoped that continuities between various themes in modernity and various psychologies/theologies will become more obvious as we proceed. From the many themes in modernity apparent in the description above, I will select several but focus on the first: pluralism, secularism, technology, and capitalism. Individualism is another obvious theme in modernity, but it will be discussed in a later chapter.

Pluralism

Modernity as a culture has many plots or themes and many storytellers, each with their own version of the grander story. There are even contradictions. Some storytellers focus on the secularity of science and technology while the others focus on the rise of a range of religious groups. Different psychological theories and therapies reflect different dimensions of the grander cultural story. Some theories may even contain the contradictions because they represent various stories.

Those societies that see themselves as modern are ones that also see themselves as pluralistic, heterogeneous. Society becomes a kaleidoscope of cultures, communities, and traditions. Each of these groups has its own story, its own set of moral obligations, its own symbol system. Each may be distinguished from other groups by language, clothing, religious expression, rituals, and sometimes social class. The ethos is cosmopolitan.

Ethnic pluralism in the West is a product of migration. The attraction to a better way of life or to religious and civil liberties has created cultures that are incredibly diverse. In the city in which I live (Fresno, California) there are 70 different ethnic groups. Teachers report that there are still 50 spoken languages represented by their students. Such is the nature of the modern society.

Psychology

The nondirective nature of some contemporary therapies is a reflection of the social force of pluralism in modernity. The therapist's rationale for neutrality is, in part, because of the plurality of values in culture and in the counseling room. If respect for diversity holds in society, it should hold in counseling as well. It is also assumed that the client already possesses the ethical resources and must learn to assume responsibility for action. When neither client nor therapist know the community of the other, then therapy becomes a relationship between a socially isolated client and a neutral, tolerant therapist. To be directive is to impose one's values. Pluralism is thus reinforced. That may well be a gift of pluralism in modernity.

However, the awareness of the plurality creates a new experience for the modern person. He or she is now aware of other and competing ideologies, values, and practices. The nemesis of cultural and religious pluralism is fragmentation. What is needed is something that creates unity and coherence. Whether in research, therapy, religion, or ethics, in each case there is a search for that which is more universal to compensate for the fragmenting impact of pluralism. The science of psychology or the principles of ethics are often treated as universal symbol systems that can provide some of that coherence to our understanding of the individual.

Introductory psychology texts in the West describe behavioral "laws" as if they are universal regardless of ethnic community, social class, or culture. Standard textbooks of psychology provide standardized ways of viewing and creating the psyche. One way in which this standardization is accomplished is through a commitment to science. It is less subjective, more reliable, and more universal than the common sense of particular ethnic communities. It is an advance over the provincialism of traditional societies. Common sense explanations and superstition are tested by systematic research. The discipline prides itself on its status as a science in contrast to less rigorous and more speculative disciplines. Traditional meanings are translated into the scientific symbol system. Learning research then focuses on processes, not the substance of what is learned, using traditionless content-nonsense syllables. Such knowledge comports well with the modern world.

Most modern psychologists tend neither to see their subject as historical nor their discipline as occurring within the context of history. The natural science model of psychology assumes the fundamental stability of behavior and relationships over time and space. Laws of psychophysics should hold in 1874 and 2001, among European Caucasians and African-Americans. It is possible that the study of human behavior in a scientific manner is possible at the biological level, where the genetic contribution is significant, and at the environmental level when the latter is so overdetermined as to consistently condition human behavior. At the level of personality, family, group, or ethnic community, predictability is virtually impossible. The presentation of personality and social behavior as patterned and lawful may then be a form of cultural imposition on traditional cultures.

While there is a legitimate place for a descriptive, empirical, scientific understanding of human phenomena, scientific psychology is also a way of socializing its believers into modernity. It does so by assuming that all its findings universally apply to human nature, thus making culture irrelevant. Psychology becomes ideological at the point at which its practitioners attribute the same stability found in biologically influenced behavior to personality and social behavior. The ideology of scientific objectivity is then a cloak for protecting Western culture. But self-reflexivity makes a predictive science of human behavior almost impossible.

Gergen (1973, 1982) has made the point that experimental findings are interpretable only against the background of a community of language users whose vocabulary and meanings correspond to those of the researchers. Clearly, an ethnic group could object that its meanings are different from those of the middle-class, Anglo-European researcher. A psychologist is actually one who creates a language to describe reality, and in so doing creates that social reality.

John Lee (1984) has raised concerns regarding the ways in which psychological ideology interacts with pluralism in the context of therapy. He has pointed to the scientific methodology of psychology as a form of cultural imposition. For many an ethnic group with such an epistemology is fundamentally alien. Together with many other psychologists, Lee is concerned that psychological inventories tend to minimize differences between cultural groups. The meaning of assertiveness and dominance, for example, varies in significant ways among ethnic groups.

Lee indicates further that the delivery and practice of counseling is encapsulated in Anglo-American perspectives. Ethnic groups tend to have their own unique understanding of the nature of illness and skills for bringing about healing. Consistent with the thrust of this chapter, Lee maintains that counseling is a modern institution. Modernity provides the helping professional with new definitions of personal fulfillment in contrast to more traditional ethnic understandings. Lee comments that "American counseling is an institution created to meet the problem of individual identity and direction in pluralistic society. Our profession, not just our techniques and theories, is a cultural institution founded on and thus reflective of our cultural beliefs and values. Our profession is a fruit of our modernity" (1984:595).

Religion

In the West we began the shift toward pluralism with the dissolution of the Medieval area. The latter was an epoch born of the Constantinian vision for a Christian society. Dissension was not tolerated. The Reformation served to create a major break in the unity of an older era. That resulted in a fundamental division between Protestant and Catholic. The process of further pluralization was encouraged by every group that sought religious liberty for its particular convictions. The Anabaptists, for example, rejected the Constantinian union of church and state and the right of the state to require the church to baptize infants. Thus the further support of religious pluralism.

When pluralism is a threat, we tend to retreat into the security of a common ideology. In the United States there is a powerful story that has shaped its ideals, its character, and its direction. Sociologists of religion call it "civil religion." The story is invoked with utmost seriousness at presidential inaugurations. The plot of the story is as follows. The American society emerged as the New Israel. We left slavery in Egypt (read British hegemony), crossed the Jordan (Atlantic), and passed into the promised land God has given us. Such a story provides an interpretation of the past, a coherent memory, some heroes, some dominant metaphors and symbols, and a direction for action. For those citizens who accept this cultural story as their own, to invoke it has a powerful impact. The therapist or preacher who references the story as a part of the therapeutic process or a sermon is no different than presidents who do the same. The story conjures up images that have potent emotional associations, and they include some prescriptions for action. If they fought for freedom, so must we. The story of civil religion is to serve as social glue and to fend off the fragmentation that comes with pluralism.

Modern pluralism has had its impact on ethics as well. MacIntyre (1981) maintains that a stable social setting creates a coherent moral discourse. In his seminal book *After Virtue,* he states that a moral philosophy presupposes a sociology. In classical societies morality and social structure are one and the same, "For every moral philosophy offers explicitly or implicitly at least a partial conceptual analysis of the relationship of an agent to his or her reasons, motives, intentions and actions, and in so doing generally presupposes some claim that these concepts are embodied or at least can be in the real social world" (1981:22). Moral language, to be understood and operative, needs a cultural context in which it is embodied. Given the pluralistic nature of modernity and the loss of community, we now possess a variety of disembodied moral languages. Given this plethora of communally homeless moral languages, MacIntyre has argued that our current moral language is fragmentary and inconsistent. The unified historical context that once gave moral propositions their meaning is now gone. In the modern world there appears no way of obtaining moral consensus. The moral terms used made sense in the particular culture in which they emerged, but debate between rival claims is interminable because there is a fundamental difference in the meaning assigned to the moral terms of the debate. Further analysis of these fragments will not result in a coherent moral language. While we continue to use moral language, MacIntyre maintains that we have largely lost our ability to engage in meaningful moral debate.

Given the absence of historical context for moral claims, the latter are presented in an ahistorical, impersonal, and abstract mode. Moral concepts and language become meaningless when they persist beyond or are wrested from the larger totalities of theory and practice in which they were accepted. In the original context one could give a rational explanation for an objective standard that was meaningful to the community. When moral ideas must in some way be justified, we have a symptom that points to the fact that the moral community, which supports the moral language, is disintegrating. When moral ideals are vital because one can systematize them or generalize them as abstract principles, one can be assured that a moral community is being assumed that is in agreement about the substance of an acceptable morality and that completes the content of the formal morality. Moral language is a linguistic residue of earlier practices of a particular moral community. *Unless* one recreates in every generation a voluntary, moral community with a voluntary confession of a particular moral ideal, moral language becomes a mere linguistic trapping.

There is in pluralistic, modern societies little consensus on moral ideals, and those that continue to exist are perceived as either arbitrary or a matter of personal preference. In the therapeutic process itself there will then be no consensus on the meaning of moral terms. When moral ideals are referenced, it is perceived as moralism. Therapy then turns to a concern with more opportunities for new experience rather than the development of common values. A healing culture has a coherent moral language. But when the social entity that supports this language disintegrates, as it has in modernity, we are left with linguistic fragments alone.

To begin with the Reign of God means that this is the criterion for testing the pluralism of modernity that affects both Christianity and culture, psychology and faith. This does not mean an uncritical acceptance or rejection of pluralism. To seek first the Reign of God means that we must choose that in culture which is consistent with the Reign of God. To affirm that the Reign of God has cultural manifestations is to recognize that there are many cultures. The Reign of God does require one to choose which cultural vision has priority. It sensitizes one to the importance of recognizing that cultures provide meaning for individuals and that one's research or therapy must respect that plurality.

The gift of religious pluralism demands respect for the differentness of worldview and ethos of other ethnic and religious groups. A commitment to the Reign of God as ethical culture is not a commitment to a return to "cultural Constantinianism." It does not assume that religion must be the glue that makes modern pluralistic societies cohere, whether its citizens so choose or not. Implicit in some conservative religious movements is such a Constantianian impulse. Conservative religious psychologists have assumed that a national policy on the family from a Christian point of view would increase the health of the American family. It might, but if it is imposed, I do not think it will. Such an approach violates the voluntarism implicit in an ethic of the Reign of God.

Secularism

Traditional societies have tended to be more religious in their worldviews while modern societies have largely embraced a secular worldview. Secularization is the process by which nature and human nature, previously perceived as religious, are no longer seen as such (Fenn, 1978). Secularists take seriously the distinction between sacred and secular. The argument of contemporary sociologists of religion is that the process of secularization is shrinking the number of behaviors traditionally perceived as religious. In other words, there are certain areas of public life that are not to be interpreted in religious terms. The secular world is the world of pure rationality. It is a world without a particular, normative story. The person in the secular world is the person released from the ancient sacred traditions. It is not a universe whose order is derived from the transcendent.

Clearly, American psychology sees itself as secular in ways consistent with the ethos of modernity. Psychologists can unwittingly be a part of this process of secularization in any number of ways.

1. Few introductory textbooks of psychology discuss religion as a topic of research.
2. When religion is a topic of discussion it is filtered through a scientific frame of reference.
3. By focusing their discipline on the study of the individual to the exclusion of the social context, psychologists reinforce a tendency toward secularization.
4. To the extent that psychologists in the therapeutic process make reference only to a linear logic that excludes the role played by tradition, symbol, and story, to that

extent they support the process of demythologizing religious convictions.

It is interesting that it is precisely cultures emerging out of Judaism that have assumed that every area of life is to be imbued by a central confession. Perhaps, then, one of the tasks of the contemporary Christian therapist is to assist in the resacralization of the client's world. Therapy can be a collaborative process in which the therapist and client reinterpret the world again through the eyes of faith.

The model of religious culture that was described in the previous chapter assumes a high degree of integration between personal and social systems of value and religiosity, so that religiosity can be applied to a wide array of behaviors, situations, rituals, and institutions in society. Thus, that which is sacred is not limited to that which is private, or to particular events, persons, places, times, or objects. The theme of the Reign of God assumes that what is needed is a sacralization of all of life. What is necessary for effectiveness of psychologists as therapists, researchers, and teachers is not simply professional competency, but the sacralization of culture in itself.

Technology

Out of the implicit metaphors and logic of science emerges the power of a technological culture (Morgan, 1968). The basic metaphor of the machine is implicit in the scientific endeavor. With a machine metaphor one can analyze problems in terms of basic components. The construction of the machine is rational and logical. The procedures for running it are standardized. The results are practical and reliable. Science follows a similar pattern. There is little room for mystery or spontaneity. Thus the model that science builds assumes that knowledge is objective rather than subjective. The relationships between variables is causal rather than dialectical. The operations of significant variables is assumed to be measurable in time and space. Laws are assumed to be invisible and universal.

The technological nature of contemporary Western society has been carefully described by Ellul (1964): technological society tends to be pragmatic, efficient, and means-oriented. Technology adopts the machine metaphor in the way it shapes culture. As a paradigm it shapes culture much the way the concept of "God" has in the past. It is oriented toward efficiency. Means are more important; ends are assumed given. Thus we are relieved of the responsibility for careful ethical discernment. Ethical problems are translated into questions of strategy. The categorical imperative or technology is that "If it can be done, it will be done."

Skinner's (1971) proposal for a technology of behavior change in many ways reflects the larger social commitment to a technological way of life. His self-proclaimed goal was to develop a technology of behavior change that is simple and efficient, and he opens his classic *Beyond Freedom and Dignity* with the hope for a technology of behavior. The presuppositions and methodological commitments of behaviorist psychology can be summarized by such adjectives as operational, mechanistic, deterministic, predictive, and positivistic. A society that values efficiency and practicality will find such an approach consistent with its own ideals. It need only be shaped by our knowledge of the laws of conditioning. Skinner engages in little discussion of ends and the nature of the good individual or the good society.

MacIntyre (1981) makes the comment that therapists in a technological society are incapable of ethical reflection. The fundamental therapeutic task is now that of efficiently adapting individuals to existing culture. The ends are given; only the means need to be selected and manipulated.

The critique of a technological society and a technological psychotherapy from a Reign of God perspective is not simply the rejection of means, of pure pragmatism. Method is not primary. Taking the Reign of God seriously means that some ends will be severely critiqued, if not rejected, and others will be affirmed. From the perspective of the Reign of God, it is not simply effectiveness that determines what needs to be done. There is a place for an ethic of faithfulness in the absence of results. A paradigm that focuses obsessively on the visible needs to recognize the fundamental mystery of God.

Capitalism

In contrast to the highly relational economic systems of traditional societies, the modern world can be described as a marketplace of impersonal transactions (Weber, 1930). Relationships

between individuals are characterized primarily by an exchange
of goods and services for fees. Therapy in such a setting may well
take on the character of an exchange of fees for friendship.
Schoefield (1964) has argued that professional counseling is
often a purchase of friendship. The moral neutrality and emotional detachment of the psychoanalyst from the patient may
also be seen as a reflection of the distance between individuals
in a market society. Moscovici (1972) suggests that American
research on small groups in social psychology assumes that
social relations are in part transactions based on rational calcu-
lation of reward and punishment. Such an orientation coincides
with relationships of a market society.

Given its industrial context, American psychology is at times
obsessed with problem solving. Decades ago, Watson (1913), in
"Psychology as the Behaviorist Views It," asserted that "if psychology would follow the plan I suggest, the educator, the
physician, the jurist, and the businessman could utilize our
data in a practical way, as soon as we are able, experimentally,
to obtain them" (160). Buss (1979) has argued that the individual differences movement and the corresponding testing indus-
try emerged with the rise of a complex division of labor common to modern societies.

In the area of developmental psychology, Klaus Riegel
(1972) described two traditions that have shaped us: the learning tradition and the organismic approach. The learning tradition came from a pragmatic cultural climate that emphasized
competition, quantitative growth, and a single standard of
evaluation (achievement-oriented intelligence tests). This tradition has predominated in capitalistic societies. The organismic approach, on the other hand, emerged out of less industrial
societies. It emphasized qualitative growth models, human
equality, and multigenerational and multicultural standards.

If capitalism and the ethic of the Reign of God do not conflict, then a psychology that reflects capitalism is a gift, not
suspect. However, if there are points of tension, then the
promise of the social sciences must at least be qualified. When
capitalism reduces therapy to a cash exchange, a business
enterprise, or the purchase of friendship, then there is clearly a
conflict. When therapy is limited to those with capital, then
again there is a conflict with an ethic that takes seriously a
commitment to the poor. If a research program deals only with

the problems raised in a capitalist culture, then the ethic of the Reign of God might suggest different research priorities.

Psychology and Culture as Ethical

Psychological theories are reflections not only of social forces, but also of the ethical nature of culture generally. In the previous chapter I made the case that culture is not neutral, it is ethical in nature. If psychological theory and practices are reflections of culture, then they are implicitly religious and ethical in nature. This is a point made some time ago by Paul Vitz (1977) and more recently by Don Browning (1988b). In his book *Religious Thought and the Modern Psychologies,* Browning uncovers the ethical and metaphysical horizons of various contemporary theories of therapy and anthropology. He does so by isolating the critical metaphors and the principles of *obligation* implicit in psychological ideology. Browning posits that

> significant portions of modern psychologies and especially clinical psychologies, are actually instances of religio-ethical thinking. They are, in fact, mixed disciplines which contain examples of religious, ethical and scientific language. To state this about the modern psychologies is certainly to go against their own self-understanding. They see themselves as sciences, and some certainly do achieve this status more completely than others. But when many of these psychologies are submitted to careful analysis one discovers that they have religious and moral horizons about which both they and the general public are unclear (1986:8).

Browning describes four cultures implicit in modern psychologies: a) a culture of detachment (Freud) perceives the world primarily in pessimistic terms; b) a culture of joy (Jung and the humanists) view the world as basically harmonious; c) a culture of control (Skinner) understands the individual as manipulated by various environments; and d) a culture of care (Erikson, Kohut) emphasizes self-transcendence and love for the other.

Modern psychologies offer us theories that tell us what we naturally want and need. The healthy person is one who has access to and control over what is needed. Psychologists provide us with developmental schedules that regulate what we need at different stages of our lives. Browning asks of any theory what fundamental needs or tendencies should be morally satisfied. Freud (id), Jung (individuation), Rogers (self-actualization), and Erikson (epigenetic development) all assume that there are needs that must be satisfied. These needs, Browning suggests, must be placed in a moral context.

Given a commitment to the ethic of the Reign of God, it is not simply a psychological theory that will determine *de facto* the language and values that shape therapy. Psychological theory and therapeutic culture are religious in nature in ways little different from most religious cultures. Psychology cannot then prescribe for other religious traditions how needs are to be prioritized or expressed. Clinical psychologies cannot escape being religious. Clients expect, and the healing process demands an ethical framework. In a pluralistic culture, the secular clinician needs to recognize that his or her ethical framework is not more legitimate because of a scientific, transhistorical foundation. It is open to the same critique as any other religion culture.

Ethics, Culture, and Psychology

The above contextualization of psychological approaches in modernity is suggestive rather than definitive. Though the relationship needs much more thorough analysis, I would submit several implications that merit attention for those concerned about the use of psychological theory, research, or practice in the Christian community. First, if knowledge and healing are functions of the quality of society, then clearly the question of what constitutes the "good society" is raised. Conflict between Christianity and psychology may emerge when the theory of the "good society" implicit in modern psychology is not consistent with the social vision of the Reign of God. Second, a commitment to the Reign of God as the "good society" demands a systematic critique and evaluation of the host culture of the church. Third, to the degree that modern culture and psychology are uncritically identified with the Reign of God, psychology and theology will serve as agents to socialize the Church into modernity. Fourth, the dialogue of faith and discipline of psychology must include a critique of culture and the church, and reflect an ethic consistent with the Reign of God.

1. A sociology of psychological knowledge logically raises the question of the nature of the "good society." If knowledge reflects society, then cultures that are oppressive, decadent, impersonal, or violently aggressive would possess a knowledge base that reflects and creates these characteristics. Conversely, the just society creates and is sustained by knowledge that is emancipatory. But the critical question is, "What constitutes the good society?" Such a definition would enable us to develop criteria for the selection of psychological insights and practices consistent with that formulation. We have suggested that in the theme of the Reign of God we have the seeds for the good society.

If modernity is synonymous with our definition of the ideal society, then there would be no conflict in the utilization of modern psychological theories and practices in moving conservative church members into the ethos of modernity. However, if one seeks a definition of the nature of the good society from a Reign of God perspective, then one might seek to develop a conception of the good society consistent with a New Testament characterization of the Reign of God. Such a culture, we are told, seeks peace, acts justly, and displays compassion. It values servanthood and faithfulness. It is the responsibility of the Church to discern what these ethical convictions will mean in our day. The highest agenda for the church that seeks to reflect the values of the Reign of God is to determine what it means to be "in the world but not of the world." Only then will we be able to test the consistency of our psychological contributions to the advancement of the Reign of God against some standard. Only when there is some consensus about the shape of such a social project can the psychologist bring to bear information, experience, and insight that is truly a contribution.

2. Given a commitment to the incarnation of the ethic of the Reign of God in society, we have a basis for an evaluation of society and the life of the church. Our response to modernity and psychology need not be one of simple rejection. Rather, a careful discernment of what is consistent or inconsistent with the ethic of the Reign of God is needed. An understanding of the Reign of God as an ethical culture makes a critique of

American psychology possible. If psychology reflects the best and worst of modernity, a systematic process of social criticism is a prerequisite. And, if we view with ambivalence the contribution of modernity, then we hope that a more discerning stance toward modern psychology as a discipline will emerge. The following assessment is illustrative of the analysis that is needed.

Pluralism allows each community its own integrity but the price is the loss of common moral language and global cultural identity. Pluralism in therapy can be simply a justification for any point of departure for worldview, ethic, or personal identity. Modernity is then a mixed blessing.

A secularism in psychology that precludes trust in God's faithfulness and presence in history, or a technological worldview that slights the importance of mystery and miracle, undermines the presence of the Reign of God on earth. Secularism has liberated us from superstition but eliminated a sense of the transcendent. Technology has increased the efficiency of production but it has also increased our sense of alienation from nature, others, self, and God. The inability of many psychological theories of change to deal creatively with authority makes impossible an ethic of joyful obedience to the law of Christ.

Capitalism has given us access to incredible resources but it has also profoundly affected the therapeutic process. A capitalism that reduces therapeutic relationships to fees for services rendered is a violation of the sacrificial ethic of the New Testament. The Enlightenment trust in rationality fails to appreciate the importance of image and symbol in religious development.

Needless to say, this summary of the interplay of the Reign of God and a critique of modernity is very preliminary. This chapter is intended only as a sketch to illustrate the connection between society, psychology, and religious perspectives.

3. If it is the case that North American psychology is in part an expression of Western ideals, it may also be the case that those who uncritically employ psychological theories and techniques in Christian therapy, pastoral counseling, Christian education, or evangelism are socializing the Christian community into the modern world in a way little different from cul-

ture-blind psychologists in Chile (Zuniga, 1975). The socializing impact of psychology could make the vision of the Reign of God indistinguishable from Western society. If we employ psychological knowledge unself-consciously, the next generation of believers might support pluralism, secularism, technicism, and capitalism uncritically.

However, the church is itself not immune to critique. Quite independent of psychological influences, the church may have absorbed the ethos of modernity as well. Needless to say, integration of psychology and Christianity under circumstances where the church is wholly acculturated is no creative task. Since both are cut from the same cloth it should come as no surprise that the two have the same texture. Critique is appropriately directed to the life of the church and to psychological practices.

The seduction of psychology as ideology is facilitated by the existence of Christian communities obsessed with boundary maintenance rather than motivated by mission. Ossified church communities can create the conditions of disaffection from the church and seduction by psychological ideologies rather than fostering a climate of thoughtful discernment. When there is no central confession that orders the life of the community, psychology as ideology fills the vacuum. When a Christian community cannot provide forgiveness and nurture, other communities will. When church communities are defensive about the creative potential of the individual, the psychological community will provide considerable reinforcement for such creativity. If the church does not have the ability to invite ultimate loyalty to the Reign of God, other loyalties will be developed.

4. While the evaluation and interpretation of psychological knowledge and therapy must occur in the context of real life communities, it might nonetheless be useful to speculate what kind of psychology would be most consistent with the ethic of the Reign of God. If the Reign of God is social in nature, then a tradition-sensitive psychology and psychotherapy seems more relevant. If the agenda of a host culture is to create social and historical change, then a deterministic psychology insensitive to change would be irrelevant if not subversive. How useful is a deterministic psychology that assumes that human nature does not change? If the Reign of God is such that its very existence

creates conflict in culture, how useful is a psychology that does not tolerate or understand the important role of conflict? Psychologists have too often focused on steady states and equilibrium rather than on the conflicts that generate change. Mental health professionals who are genuinely concerned about the development of a culture consistent with the Reign of God must be ready to analyze critically the consistency of the assumptions of their own psychology with the agenda of the Reign of God.

3

On Hearing
and Telling Stories

If it is the case that great art or literature is creative because it has its foundation in a sustaining story or tradition, why should that not be the case with therapy as well? For other disciplines the sustaining heritage has been the panoply of Greek and Roman gods, the Medieval synthesis, the Renaissance and Reformation, the Enlightenment, or modern capitalism. I suggested in the last chapter that psychology and psychotherapy as we know them are rooted in the modern myth. This chapter will focus specifically on the therapeutic process and its relationship to story.

Among the ways a culture socializes its members into its ethos is *narrative,* the telling of stories. Stories carry implicitly the primary images, metaphors, and paradigms of a culture. The civil religion described in the last chapter is an example. An internal grammar coordinates the images and gives them coherence. The storyteller is one who by telling a story reinforces or qualifies the structure of a culture. If the storyteller, whether teacher or comedian, preacher or parent, lawyer or therapist, is legitimated by the culture, then the structure of the culture is more easily absorbed in its hearers. Stories are one way a culture creates a common worldview, an acceptable ethos, and a sense of personal identity.

Therapists "tell" stories, stories that emerge out of a particular culture. In so doing they socialize their clients into the values and worldview they have in common, a task incredibly complex given the plurality of communities in modernity. This chapter will describe the role narrative plays in therapy and again ask the question what difference it makes if we begin with the primacy of the story of the Reign of God. In this chapter, I will claim that one way in which the ethic of the Reign of God is internalized is through story. In a religious context, a person who seriously reads the Scriptures is making a story normative, a gauge for the understanding of one's personal story. Every culture has its own sacred stories that give meaning to suffering and joy, birth and death. To seek first the Reign of God is to make it our sacred story.

In Richard Adams' (1972) fascinating novel, *Watership Down,* we are given a powerful statement about the role of stories in the life of a unique culture. At one level this novel is about the sundry adventures of a wandering warren of rabbits. What is unique about rabbits, we are told, is their ability to tell stories. There is a saying among them that a rabbit "can no more refuse to tell a story than an Irishman can refuse to fight" (apparently stereotypes are operative in their world as well). Their stories define who they are and give them the skills to survive in a fragile world. They have stories of origin and stories of liberation. Some stories are told to discern new direction; some are told to reinforce the status quo. There are stories that make the community open to the stranger and there are stories that make leadership legitimate rather than arbitrary.

In their travels the rabbits visit other communities that contrast the nature of their own community. One of the warrens they encounter in their travels has no name. It also has no stories and no tradition. Its primary characteristic is that it is a warren without a chief rabbit and each rabbit does as it pleases. After the wandering group shares one of their stories, an individual in this strange warren comments: "Yes very nice . . . I always think these traditional stories retain a lot of charm, especially when told with real old-fashioned spirit." Unlike this character, Barbara Hardy suggests we are story-driven people. She states: "For we dream in narrative, daydream in narrative, remember, anticipate, hope, despair, believe, doubt, plan, revise, criticize, construct, gossip, learn, hate, and love by narrative. In order to live, we make up stories about ourselves and others, about the personal as well as the social past and future" (as quoted in Gerkin, 1986:29).

The concern of this chapter is to use the metaphor of story to build a bridge between the Reign of God as the culture and the process of therapy. As we remember from our math classes of yesteryear, fractions that do not have a common denominator need to be made comparable to simplify addition. Similarly we need a point of commonality between faith and healing. I submit that *story* is one such point of contact. Both the life and mission of the Christian and of the therapist involve narration. In therapy, whether narrative is present and which narrative is chosen is critical when we listen to the story of those we counsel, when we construct our own identity as therapists, and when we set goals for therapy. In religion, narrative is evident in the Scriptures we read, in the way our identity is shaped by normative biographies, and in the way we invite others to become part of God's story.

The Modern Context

If one examines contemporary ethics in terms of the grander plot of modernity, one can better understand the importance of a recovery of narrative. As already mentioned in a previous chapter, MacIntyre (1981) analyzes the impact of modern existence on ethics. He suggests that at issue is what has happened to the nature of moral languages and moral resources in modern societies. In short, our moral languages do not cohere and our moral resources are depleted. In our pluralist society we are left with a Babel of ethical languages. They are rooted in utilitarianism, hedonism, pragmatism, and duty. What we now possess are fragmented pieces wrested from their earlier more meaningful historical contexts (narratives) and pressed into service as part of contemporary moral discourse. What results is at best a confusing dialogue, at worst a nonconversation. In the absence of common moral discourse, moral judgments are now a matter of personal preference on the one hand or abstract generalizations on the other.

If the story that once gave a culture meaning is lost, the moral demands are experienced as oppressive. Before I examine the relationship of the Reign of God to story and therapy, I will reflect on the therapeutic process in terms of the client's story, the therapist's story, and the collaborative narrative that emerges as a result of the client-therapist relationship. I will discuss each of these in turn with the help of stories and summary statements.

Their Story

Stories in therapy tap into the structure of personal and cultural consciousness. In a seminal article Steven Crites (1971) posited that the quality of human experience is fundamentally narrative in nature. It is temporal; there is the memory of present as past and future that became present. Stories tend to mark memory, to order inchoate consciousness. Stories told by others shape consciousness because they are made of the same stuff; they are not an arbitrary imposition.

Stories are not simply charming tales told to stimulate nostalgia. Karen Lebacqz (1985) makes the case that action and the definition of motives are never separable from one's story. In the telling of my story, I give reasons for what I do. We live by the imposition of a story on the disparate events of our lives. Stories describe certain kinds of responses to situational demands. They help us to know what to look for in a situation and which features in a situation are crucial. Actions take on different meanings depending on the story used to interpret the act. It is possible that descriptions of an act are not consistent with what we know of an agent's character or story.

By our actions and cognitions we construct a story. We are known and revealed in the life-stories that emerge out of our agency. That story has temporal dimensions of past, present, and future. It depends on the cognitive functions of memory, awareness, and anticipation. The meaning of such life-stories is seen from the end point, eschatologically. Our storytelling expresses how we live. A number of psychologists (Bettelheim, 1977; Fellner, 1976; Gardner, 1971; Gordon, 1978; Harre and Secord, 1972; Hillman, 1972; Hobson, 1971; Spence, 1982) have maintained that the fundamental form of active consciousness is narrative in nature. Harre and Secord (1972) suggest a dramaturgical approach to understanding human behavior in contrast to more deterministic perspectives. To think, feel, and act is to be historical; it is to tell a story.

On the other hand, the profoundly troubled soul is unable to tell any story. Navone and Cooper argue that "the ability to organize one's memories, present reality, and future expectations, the ability to experience one's self as the single subject of a continuous narrative, in short, the ability to tell one's story, is a *sine qua non* of mental health" (1981:49).

One of the most extensive analysis of the relationship of story to therapy is provided by the work of James Hillman. He indicates: "From my perspective as depth psychologist, I see that those who have a connection with story are in better shape and have a better prognosis than those to whom story must be introduced. . . . to have 'story-awareness' is *per se* psychologically therapeutic" (1975a:1).

Hillman has commented that "one integrates life as a story because one has stories in the back of the mind (unconscious) as containers for organizing events into meaningful experiences" (1975a:1). He suggests that psychoanalysis is, first of all, to be regarded as an activity in the realm of *poesis.* He suggests that case history is a new form of literary genre. It is written at the level of the objective and real and at the level of drama and imagination. Case histories are a way of writing stories. In the case history of Dora, Freud seemed to use standard techniques of storytelling: the creation of a setting, suspense, concealment, resolution. The story begins with incoherence and moves towards coherence. These case histories are not scientific materials in the strict sense: there is no possibility of checking the results. Freud's case histories are the stuff of fiction. They express the narrative side of human nature.

The particular story of an individual is always formed in the context of a myriad of cultural myths. Different cultures have different stories and thus different ways of interpreting acts. To the extent that the cultural myths provided to the individual are coherent, the individual is helped somewhat. But there is the larger question of the content and direction of the narratives. The answer to that question must be provided by one's primary narrative.

Stories are the ways clients make their lives plausible. Clients begin therapy by telling a story, their story. It is a story that attempts to create coherence and consistency amid fragmentation and confusion. A younger female client, severely punished during adolescence, constructs the themes of her personal story around fear of authorities, hatred of her father, the unpredictability of people, security in and dependence on her spouse. A middle-aged female client, depressed for more than fifteen years, describes herself as a woman who was not allowed to construct her own personal story. It was assumed that women did not have the ability to do so. An older male relates how his father belittled his ability and how he has never forgotten it nor ever achieved anything.

Roy Shafer (1981) makes the point that troubled clients develop stories that give coherence to their actions. They construct stories that are more livable. The self-conscious articulate client comes to therapy with already formed stories that focus on the problems of the main character. Clients with only one story project that story on every sequence of events, a process usually referred to as transference.

The responsibility of any therapist is to listen attentively to the story of the troubled individual. In doing so one obtains a feel for the major characters, the nature of the plot and subplots, the probable outcome, and the relationship of the story to other stories one has heard. There are a series of questions one can have in mind when listening to a client's stories that enable one to sense the cultural context. What are the recurring themes? What is the central image? What is the feeling tone of the storyteller? What resources are implied by the story of the client? Can I use related images in a known story that will enable one to incorporate those new images that are healing? Is the story coherent? Does the story have a plot? People who seek help are often those who have no stories or have stories with no plot, who have no significant characters, or have major discontinuities in their life. Does the teller "own" the story or is it told in a passive voice? How is the personal story connected to the dominant cultural myths? Can the storyteller reflect on the story with some objectivity? What is the individual sharing, an explanation or a story?

The Therapist's Story

Therapists have a personal story. We are storytellers by the kind of people we are. Therapists are not simply problem solvers or technicians. We are not only interviewers or empathic listeners. We are not simply objective scientist-practitioners. We are not simply analysts of abstract forces at play in the lives of our clients. The kinds of stories we possess, consciously and unconsciously, shape the process of therapy. Hillman states, "the way we tell our story is the way we form our therapy. The way we imagine our lives is the way we are going to live our lives" (1975b:53). This issue will receive major attention in Part 3.

Therapists bring to bear their assumptions regarding the nature of good plots. Donald Spence (1982) has argued that the psychoanalyst is an archeologist. What a therapist does is to engage in an active process of constructing a plausible story of the client's past. Shafer (1981) suggests that Freud operated on the basis of two primary plots in reconstructing a client's past. Each of the stories became a standard, a way of interpreting the stories of clients. They have become normative plots. The first assumes the child is the unsocialized, instinct-driven being who must be tamed by civilization. If the process goes well, the child moves from irrational helplessness and domination by instincts to stability, mastery, rationality, and security. The second Freudian narrative is based on Newtonian physics and views the psyche as machine. The psyche is then viewed in terms of inertia; one is moved by forces, and love is seen in terms of the displacement and utilization of energy. Balance in the system is achieved through defense mechanisms.

While Freud was a writer *of* fictions in terms of case material, Jung was a writer *on* fictions. Though Jung did not accept Freud's fiction of the dream, he did in fact regard the dream as a manifestation of the gods. The dream for Jung was metaphorical; for Freud it was allegorical. The allegorical approach assumes latent and manifest material and requires translation of one into the other. The metaphorical mode for Jung is the very voice of culture within. The symbolic structure is part of the structure of human nature. Thus, if psychotherapists wish to understand the dreaming soul, they must turn to a different logic.

Freud's plots for therapy are simple. They involve repression, followed by excitement and conflict, the involvement of the therapist-author, the reduction of the repression through new recognitions, and the denouement of therapy. Jung charged that Freud's scheme was too simplistic—i.e., his plots were too simple. Jung assumed the intentionality of characters and focused not simply on causality. Freud seemed to focus entirely on narrative with only one plot. Jung's plots are multiple and variegated.

To summarize, the plot of a story reveals human intentions. It is what makes a story cohere, make sense. A story answers what happens next, while the plot tells us why. In case histories the plots are our theories. Simple theories are referred to as parsimonious; simple plots are called elegant. It is through stories (in part) that the impact of a culture is made or brought to bear on the therapeutic process. Psychologists, pastoral counselors, and social workers are mandated storytellers. By what they say and do they reinforce the larger culture story. Their accumulated knowledge and wisdom is born in the context of a culture and in turn reinforces that culture.

Our Story

From a narrative perspective, the goal of therapy is the emergence of a better story. While walking the hospital grounds Milton Erickson once encountered a patient who indicated that he was indeed Jesus Christ. Without addressing the delusion, Erickson began a meandering conversation that included references to carpentry. After some time he inquired whether the patient had any woodworking skills. Yes indeed he did. Would he be willing to make something for him, Erickson inquired. He would. Erickson requested he make him a very simple construction. Some days later when the patient had completed the task, Erickson increased the level of difficulty. Eventually the patient constructed very finely crafted furniture, was discharged from the hospital, and went into business for himself. The delusion vanished. What Erickson did therapeutically was to take seriously the story that shaped this client's life and creatively use one of its critical images to move toward healing (Wilk, 1985).

While patients may tell their stories, the sensitive clinician reinterprets the purpose and monitors the way stories are told. With an eye for the pathological, the therapist constructs a diagnostic story; it is usually a literal, factual history, but nonetheless a creative act of writing. The client then begins to reshape his or her life into the shape of a story co-constructed with a therapist. The goal of therapy for Shafer (1981) is to enable the individual to be aware of the self as a story creator. Truth begins with the realization that we are story creators. Some stories are blatantly destructive, such as the story that assumes the victim of sexual abuse is responsible for the abuse. That story requires redefinition.

Therapy is a way of helping counselees construct new stories or revive imagination so they can exercise their ability to create different narratives themselves. Such therapy picks up again the oral tradition of telling stories. Hillman states: "Therapy is a restorying of life. Therapy is not simply the trimming of imagination and bringing it into the service of realistic goals. Therapy as story moves us from the fiction of reality to the reality of fiction. Perhaps people go to therapy to be told a soul story and give them a plot to live by" (Hillman, 1975b:57).

A story can provide greater coherence and self-knowledge. The therapist may challenge the themes of the counselee's story and be rejected. The confrontation is a breakdown in the thematic motif; the events in the client's story no longer hold together. The patient must search for a new story. Sometimes the client is without a plot and needs a new story, while at other times the individual has a story that needs reimagining. Some stories have not been plumbed for their hermeneutic possibilities, their covert meanings. Often the stories are taken too literally. In the case of Dora, Freud took her story and gave it a new plot. Hillman suggests that "successful therapy is thus a collaboration between fictions, a revisioning of the story into a more intelligent, more imaginative plot, which also means a sense of mythos in all the parts of the story" (1975b:89).

In a pluralistic culture the stories are many, and all stories are considered legitimate. The process of fashioning a meaningful story occurs not only in specific relationships, but also in the host culture. Culture *is* a story, *has* a story, and *provides* a story. Cultures provide stories that mark the memory of a people. They retell the origins, battles, ideals, and prejudices in the form of a story. In the process of telling their stories, cultures socialize each successive generation.

Hillman suggests it is time to recognize the important role fiction plays in psychotherapy and to enrich our repertoire of stories. The most common narratives are the following: epic (ego's development despite obstacles and defeat), comic (happy end despite bumbling inadequacies), detective (tracking down symptoms), and social realism (factual case histories.) The story of a client can be read in terms of these four genres. Hillman suggests that therapy may be most helpful when a person is able to place his or her life within this variety.

However, in a pluralist culture, as indicated in the last chapter, each community has a story and is legitimate. The therapist is faced with this plurality in the context of therapy. Are all stories truly equal? Are there no criteria by which to assess stories?

A Narrative Christianity

There are those for whom religion is primarily propositional, a systematic ordering of thought. The Christian life is lived according to a rational theology—consistent, coherent, and comprehensive. It is communicated best through sermons on the printed page. On the other hand, recently there have been a number of theologians who suggest that narrative is an appropriate form of expression of our faith (Crossan, 1975; Gerkin, 1984, 1986; Goldberg, 1982; McFague, 1975). In fact there are those who suggest that without story, ethics and theology become arid.

If story is the structure of personal reality, then philosophical and scientific approaches may well be limiting if not distorting. For Hans Frei (1982), the nature of the biblical literature is narrative and mirrors human reality and experience. Similarly, for Sallie McFague (1975), the structure of reality and the nature of biblical truth are metaphorical. Jesus is the parable of God. However, my assertion is *not* that the narrative nature of human experience is the justification for seeing the Reign of God as narrative, that ontology is the basis of ethics. Rather, the narrative nature of human experience is the form to which the Reign of God gives meaningful content.

The theological ethicist, Stanley Hauerwas (1977, 1981), has maintained that what we need is a different way of perceiving the moral self. He suggests that the coherence of our moral lives is tied to how we perceive the world and that the way we see the world is in turn shaped by the stories we adopt as our own. This is a more historical way of viewing the self. He states,

> Narrative is the characteristic form of our awareness of our-selves as historical beings who must give an account of the pur-posive relation between temporally discrete realities. Indeed the ability to provide such an account, to sustain its growth in a liv-ing tradition, is the central criterion for identifying a group of people as a community. Community joins us with others to fur-ther the growth of a tradition whose manifold story lines are meant to help individuals identify and navigate the path to the good. The self is subordinate to the community rather than vice versa, for we discover the self through a community's narrated tradition (1977:28).

The Old Testament is replete with examples of how stories shape culture. In fact, the Israelites are expected to tell the story to their children as they walk, as they eat, or whenever the opportunity presents itself (Deut. 6:1–6). Their rituals were condensed stories. The passover, for example, recounted the story of the Exodus. The Reign of God is not simply a catalogue of ethical demands. It is quintessentially ethical, but ethical injunction is often framed within the context of a story, the story of how and in what direction God is forming a people. Ethics is not simply a matter of applying rules to particular sit-uations. Rules within the Christian framework cannot be divorced from the narrative context. The Decalogue, for exam-ple, is a part of the covenant of God with Israel that includes their liberation from oppression and new life in a new land. Christian ethics need not begin by emphasizing rules or princi-ples but could begin by calling our attention to a narrative that tells of God's dealing with creation. Hauerwas states: "Story is fundamental to the way we talk of God. Narrative is crucial for knowledge of self, God and the world. From a religious per-spective, we know who we are when we can locate our stories within God's story" (1977:27).

A distinction is often made between a sign and a symbol. A sign is a representation of a known entity while a symbol is a formulation of something unknown. Since the Reign of God was unknown to Jesus' hearers he pointed to it through stories and comparisons. Symbols spark our imagination and motivate us to move in a particular direction. Metaphors also have a tropic function. Tropic refers to a literary technique whereby we break open our conception and perceptual fixes so that we see reality more clearly. It is the "ah hah" experience. Symbols are multideterminant in their meanings. Thus when one fixes an interpretation the symbol is reduced to a sign.

Narrative Christianity and Healing

The biblical story of the Reign of God is not simply a story available to satisfy the human need for coherent narrative. The Christian tradition assumes it is a story with a plot that can bring healing, with characters that are changed by God's presence, and with a theme that is more just. James Ashbrook (1987) talks of the biblical story as our "language of origin," "our native language," "our inheritance," "our prized possession," and "our special giftedness." He makes the assumption that the biblical story is relevant for all humanity. As the individual story is contextualized in the biblical story it is lifted into universal experience. Our story becomes a part of God's story. That, in part, is the nature of therapy.

The role of story in therapy is not simply a matter of quoting Scripture. Narrative plays a critical role in therapy when a therapist lifts up and uses the metaphors a client brings, when he or she connects them to symbols in the larger human community and, where appropriate, to the biblical story. When metaphors and themes consistent with the Reign of God emerge naturally in the therapeutic conversation it would be appropriate for the therapist who seeks first the Reign of God to recognize them as such, and to draw out their implications and connections to the deep structure of the human soul. With a religious client, one can point to the Father God who transcends abusive human fathers. The God who takes us under wings as a mother hen is not the same as an overprotective manipulative mother. The plot of crucifixion and resurrection can be related to the story of despair at the death of one's prospective bride. The experience of the Israelites can be connected to the life story of the poor and oppressed in our day. The story of the Reign of God reinterprets and shapes experience in terms of our collective Christian memory. Its parables, metaphors, and plot translate a client's one-dimensional reality into multidimensional perspectives. Ashbrook states: "In short, a judicious use of our language of origin, even when it must be taught, and mostly we are required to teach it to our clients, even as other therapists are required to teach their clients their mythologies, transforms a fixed frame of meaning into a reframing of renewing realities. In our jargon, we call that 'metanoia,' a turning around to move in a liberating direction" (1987:13–14).

One of the examples of the healing nature of the Christian story is the experience of William Kurelek (1973). Born in 1927 to poor immigrant farmers in northern Alberta, Canada, Kurelek developed feelings of depression and helplessness. His father had hoped that he would become a doctor, but he became instead an introspective and sensitive artist. After undergraduate studies at the University of Manitoba and a period of wandering through Mexico and the United States, Kurelek sought psychotherapeutic help at Maudsley Hospital in London, England. He began portraying his childhood traumas on canvas. In a painting entitled "The Maze," Kurelek depicted his body in fetal position, lying on the prairie. His brain, sawn open, is an exitless maze. Each chamber is an anxiety-ridden childhood memory. In one chamber Kurelek is feeling rejected by his playmates. Another portrays his fear of abandonment by his father. In yet another he depicts himself as caught between his smiling and angry father. In a painting entitled, "I spit on life," Kurelek reasoned that "If there is no God, no after life, no final justice, then suicide is really quite reasonable" (Kurelek, 1973:42).

The dancing classes at Maudsley Hospital were for Kurelek a senseless merry-go-round. The psychiatric panel was an ordeal and the doctors were a conspiracy. It was an occupational therapist, Margaret Smith, who befriended Kurelek. Upon discovering that she was Catholic, Kurelek began studying Catholicism. After several attempts at suicide, further psychotherapy, and electroconvulsive shock treatment, Kurelek was released. He attributed his eventual recovery to his acceptance of the Christian story as his own. He says, "Christians have a name for what was happening to me. It is called *Grace.*" His subsequent art reflects his love for life and a hope for a new humanity. He ridicules the moon explorations as a waste of money and criticizes the lack of concern for the hungry in our society. His more recent work depicts the consequences of a nuclear holocaust. The relevance of Kurelek's biography for us is its simple reminder that the Christian story has created a culture that has some healing resources. Further, it illustrates how therapy can lead to an ethical vision of culture.

Conclusion

I have made the claim that the theme of the Reign of God is relevant to the dialogue of faith and profession. In this section I have asserted that the Reign of God is a cultural manifestation and that as such it has implications for the way we understand modernity and psychotherapy. I have suggested that therapy needs a cultural (*qua* ethical) context and that God's mission is the creation of a just culture. The Reign of God is a world-view embedded in narrative. As such it has the potential of being a cognitive and emotional reconstruction of our perception of physical reality, human origins, life, and destiny. The fundamental questions of ignorance, pain, and injustice are addressed. It can become a fund of shared meanings embodied in symbols. As such, the Christian story can give coherence, rhythm, and unity to a people.

In the previous chapter we moved from the more abstract definition of culture to a concrete analysis of modernity as the context of therapy. Our thinking and healing does not occur in simply any culture. It occurs in the context of modernity. Western psychology and Christianity are in part shaped by modernity and it is my hope that the theme of the Reign of God would influence how we see both the discipline, the nature of our faith, and, in turn, the dialogue between them.

In this chapter, the focus was on the narrative nature of culture and of our faith. Again the move is toward greater particularity—the story of the Reign of God. The focus was not simply on any story but on one story. It is a story that has in the past been healing and can be in the future.

What are the implications for the religious therapist? Our first responsibility is to recognize our spiritual treasure. We must be completely convinced that God is in the business of creating a new social order, a new story. This is our most significant resource for therapy. For us to function out of our story is not necessarily to be moralistic and dogmatic. In a pluralistic culture the Christian story does not have the authority it did in the past.

Pluralism grants an individual the right to function within one's story if it is not arbitrarily imposed on others. Pluralism is then a gift to the religious therapist. The uniqueness and particularity of our story is then an asset, not a liability.

If we are not embarrassed with the particularity of the Christian story, then we can begin the difficult task of relating our story to other stories of healing in the modern world. I sense, however, that the church is embarrassed when comparing its story to the stories offered by the mental health profession. Mental health professionals have reminded us that Christianity has been dogmatically preached, has overwhelmed individuals with unresolved guilt, and has not taken seriously the most rejected in our society. Granted. But the fault lies not with the story. The story of the Reign of God remains a story that includes the outcast—the Gentile, the woman, the poor, the mentally, physically, and emotionally disabled. The story of the Reign of God gives dignity to the human individual as one made in the image of God. Here is a story that holds out the possibility of forgiveness, reconciliation, and restitution. No automatic connection is made between sin and disability. It is a story in which faithfulness to the counselee is encouraged when healing fails to occur.

In the next section I will examine more specifically how the church as a sign of God's people constructs the moral content of the ethical terms that emerge in therapy. The power of the story of God's people to heal emerges when it is embodied in particular, concrete, historical communities. MacIntyre (1981) has most eloquently made the case for communities that carry an alternative vision. He states,

> It is always dangerous to draw too precise parallels between one historical period and another; and among the most misleading of such parallels are those which have been drawn between our own age in Europe and North America and the epoch in which the Roman empire declined into the Dark Ages. None the less certain parallels there are. A crucial turning point in that earlier history occurred when men and women of good will turned aside from the task of shoring up the Roman *imperium* and ceased to identify the continuation of civility and moral community with the maintenance of the *imperium*. What they set themselves to achieve instead—often not recognizing fully what they were doing—was the construction of new forms of commu-

nity within which the moral life could be sustained so that both morality and civility might survive the coming ages of barbarism and darkness. If my account of our moral condition is correct, we ought also to conclude some time now we too have reached that turning point. What matters at this stage is the construction of local forms of community within which civility and the intellectual and moral life can be sustained through the new dark ages which are already upon us (1981:245).

Part 2

The Church
as Ethical Community

4

That Individual

haim Potok's (1972) riveting books, *My Name is Asher Lev* and *The Gift of Asher Lev* deal with the tension of a creative artist in a Hassidic Jewish community. As is the case in most powerful communities, this one too has a rich sense of history. Asher Lev knows his lineage back to the fifteenth century for both parents. There is a profound sense of solidarity between individuals in the community and between generations. If one person hurts, all suffer. Hence, Asher Lev's father expends a lifetime assisting European Jews in reconstructing their communities after the devastation of the second world war. There is a clear awareness of the continuity between generations. To kill a person is not simply to annihilate that individual but to destroy all successive generations.

Here is a community that is not embarrassed by the distinctiveness that emerges out of a dress code, customs, and a unique dialect—Yiddish. The result is a sense of identity among the members of the community. This is a community in which there is still legitimated authority. The rabbi commands respect. It is not arbitrary authority, for it emerges out of the consistency of the rabbi's life and the vision of the Jewish community. It is a community that has definite values, and there is considerable consensus about those values. They include respect for parents, the sanctity of life, loyalty, friendships, etc.

There is however, one thing that the community does not value—art.

Asher Lev, however, is a gifted young painter. He is deeply sensitive to texture, hue, and line. He is a precocious artist and an observant Jew. He wears a scull cap, retains his sidecurls, and recites the *Shema*. His parents cannot understand; the Rabbi does. The rabbi accepts Asher's gift and finds a mentor to nurture it. The mentor introduces Asher to the world of art. His teacher warns Asher that it is a very individualistic world where one paints personal feelings regardless of the consequences. His mentor states: "We painters are an individualistic lot. We are restless and rebellious." Asher discovers that no one can be a painter unless one is willing to leave behind all communities, to transcend all communities. One must paint the truth as one sees it. The novel closes with Asher Lev painting a picture of his mother crucified on a window frame. His parents are horrified that Asher would use the symbolism of the cross. For Jews it had been associated with so much suffering. The Rabbi asks Asher to leave the community.

The tension between the individual and the community is at the heart of this second section. With whom do we identify in Potok's novel? With the bright young artist who maintains his integrity and courageously paints his truest feelings despite incredible social pressure? Or with the parents and the community? Or with the Rabbi who seeks the welfare of the community and requests Asher to use his gift in such a way that the unity of the community is not destroyed?

In this part I wish to examine the role of the church as a sign of the Reign of God in relationship to ethics and healing. Just as the story of the Reign of God points to a culture that is ethical in nature, the church points to the Reign of God when it teaches and reflects God's story. If we refuse to be embarrassed by the particularity of the Christian story, we may have the energy to help a particular community to incarnate that story. I believe the church can be a healing community when it over-embodies a consensus about its values, develops a compelling, practical ethic, and creates a sense of accountability for the individual to the Christian community. However, a society that emphasizes individual rights makes the development of a sense of community exceedingly difficult. The Hassidic community is a moral community shaped by Jewish culture and norms. Like the Amish, in an individualistic culture it is an anomaly. Granted, the role of the individual is not understood well, but the focus in this section will be on the role of community in creating moral/ethical resources.

While in the first section I hoped to set the grander stage in terms of the vision of the Reign of God, now the concern is to explore the *concrete* implications of that ethical vision for the life of the church and for the professional therapist. The focus will be on the church as a specific historical community that is called to discern the will of God and, by its very life, to live out the confession that the Reign of God should be the highest priority.

There is at least one major obstacle the Christian community faces if it seeks to be a community of ethical discernment: individualism. Individualism undermines the church as an ethical community. Before exploring the main theme of this section, this chapter will focus on the role individualism has played in Western society and in mental health theories and practices.

The argument of this chapter is as follows: the Western contribution to an understanding and respect for individuality has degenerated into individualism. Classic liberalism holds a high view of the individual but a low view of society. When society is no longer blatantly oppressive, then the continued obsession with freedom ends in narcissism. Many a psychologist has embraced the liberal paradigm as is evident in their view of human nature, in their models of therapy, and in their psychologies of religion. A psychology that takes a sense of community seriously will be in conflict with and provide an alternative to contemporary individualist theories of identity and therapy.

The Liberal Tradition and Individuality

The history of the West can be read as one long paean of praise to the emancipated, self-aware, independent, and heroic individual. It was Socrates who first reminded us of the importance of knowing ourselves in order to live the examined life. Jesus refers to the Reign of God being in each individual. Augustine in his confessions legitimated serious introspection. Luther, in Renaissance fashion, could say, "Here I stand, I can do no other" in the face of the Roman church. And in the context of the Enlightenment these themes were given even greater prominence. In John Stuart Mill we have a statement of the political liberties of the individual, while Marx made an eloquent plea on behalf of the alienated person. Kierkegaard requested that his epitaph read "The Individual." Jacques Ellul has argued that it is Western civilization that focused attention on the individual and defended the inalienable right of the individual. "The West was the first civilization in history to focus attention on the individual and on freedom. . . . The West alone has defended the inalienable rights of the human person, the dignity of the individual. . . . The West has inspired man to demand his freedom, to take his stand in the face of society and affirm his value as an individual" (1978:17, 18). In the Liberal perspective as it emerged out of the Enlightenment, the individual assumed considerable importance (Hobhouse, 1964; Macpherson, 1962; Unger, 1975). The individual is the locus of values, decisions, and defining experiences. The individual must be emancipated from dead tradition and an oppressive society. From the Romanticism of Rousseau and Goethe and their colleagues, and from the liberal theories of John Stuart Mill and Jeremy Bentham emerges a profile of personal identity. Classic liberalism applauds the uniqueness of the person, extols autonomy, sanctifies privacy, assumes self-sufficiency, and celebrates the intrinsic dignity of the individual.

> 1. *Uniqueness.* Rousseau begins his "Confessions" with the statement, "I am made unlike anyone I have ever met; I will even venture to say that I am like no one in the whole world. I may be no better, but at least I am different" (1954:17).
>
> Uniqueness is the individuality that comes as a result of biological accident and as a consequence of one's own history of development. The uniqueness of the individual contrasts with the view of society that obliterates this distinctiveness.
>
> 2. *Autonomy.* The individual is independent. This independence is a function of the exercise of reason and choice. For Immanuel Kant morality was based on the principles that "all maxims are repudiated which cannot accord with the will's own enactment of universal law. The will is therefore not merely subject to the law, but is so subject that it must be considered as also making the law for itself and precisely on this account

as first of all subject to the law (of which it can regard itself as the author)" (quoted in Lukes, 1973:54–55). The freedom of the individual then is based on the rational will.

3. *Privacy.* Mill made explicit a distinction between public and private. He argued that the private world constituted an individual's feeling and thought world. It included one's tastes, preferences, plans, opinions, and conscience. It affects only the individual and hence the individual is sovereign over the private domain.

4. *Self-sufficiency.* Von Humboldt (Mill's mentor) proposed that the true end of the person was "the highest and most harmonious development of his powers to a complete and consistent whole" (Lukes, 1973:68). The highest ideal consisted of developing oneself from one's inmost nature and for one's own sake. Resources for personal development were to be found within the individual.

5. *Worth.* Liberalism affirms the supreme and intrinsic worth of the individual human being. Similarly, Kant argued that "man in general and every rational being, exists as an end in himself, not merely as a means for arbitrary use by this or that will: he must in all his actions, whether they are directed to himself or to other rational beings, always be viewed at the same time as an end" (Lukes, 1973:50).

The view of society implicit in the liberal perspective of the individual assumes that society is an entity separate from the person. A radical distinction is made between public and private. That separate community at best allows each person to pursue his/her own enlightened self-interest and at worst encroaches on personal freedoms. The former assumes that society is a collection of individuals bound by a social contract that allows each to develop personal interests without harming others. It provides support but it does not demand. The latter assumes that society too easily presumes authority over the individual. Institutional authority then takes precedence over personal authority. Autonomy is sacrificed and privacy eliminated. The individual simply becomes a pawn in the hands of the collectivity. The hierarchical structure of traditional societies allows some to develop at the expense of others and assumes that the individual will conform to the expectations of a particular social position. In contrast, classic liberalism takes the individual as given, assumes a positive view of human nature, and an ambivalent view toward community and society.

Individualism

While liberalism has defended the inalienable rights of the individual and has been instrumental in the emancipation of many from oppression, in the twentieth century we have moved from protecting the individual to a worship of the individual, from sanctity to idolatry, from individuality to individualism, from independence to autonomy, from self-fulfillment to narcissism, from privacy to subjectivism, from liberty to license. The individual becomes the center of all values, decisions, and significant experiences; groups or communities become negative. It makes shambles of tradition and history (Berger, 1977; Berger, Berger, and Keller, 1973; Weinstein and Platt, 1969; Wolff, 1968).

In his powerful critique of American society, Christopher Lasch (1978) has argued that liberalism has degenerated into a culture of narcissism. Western societies have created individuals who are tolerant but unable to hold convictions. They focus on individual development to the exclusion of cultural achievement. The narcissists dismiss guilt as anachronistic but live with anxiety about the meaning of life. They are liberated from superstitions and dogmas but have no overarching sense of metaphysical order. While competitive relationships are rejected, those relationships that are developed tend to be temporary. Achievement is sought, but all goals have been made equally acceptable. The self is to be clarified, not sacrificed to some ideal. Inner conflict receives more attention than social conflict. Goodwin (1974) has summarized it clearly:

> Individualism, which had its inception in the rebellion against medieval order, has culminated in an ideology that equates liberty with the absence of all bonds, all commitments, all restraints upon individual action. The ideology assumes recog-

nizable social form in the dissolution of the human connections traditionally sustained by social institutions such as the family, community, common social purposes, and accepted moral authority. . . . The ideology of individualism is so powerful that we . . . look on bonds as restraints; on values as opinions or prejudices; on customs as impositions. The remaining structures of shared existence . . . are assaulted as unjust obstacles in the way of liberty, as impediments to the free assertion of the self. The new consciousness . . . now, inevitably, suffocates human freedom (28, 60).

Lest we should assume that individualism is a recent phenomenon in America, it must be stated that only the word is new. Alexis de Tocqueville (1956) was the first to use the term to describe an individual's relationship to society. In the middle of the nineteenth century, de Tocqueville toured America and recorded his impressions in his book *Democracy in America*. He states:

They owe nothing to any man, they expect nothing from any man; they acquire the habit of always considering themselves as standing alone, and they imagine that their whole destiny is in their own hands. . . . Each person, withdrawn into himself, behaves as though he is a stranger to the destiny of all others. . . . And if on these terms there remains a sense of family, there no longer remains a sense of society (194).

Individualism, from the perspective of those committed to community, results in the loss of both the individual and of community. Emile Durkheim (1951), in his now classic study of suicide, concluded that suicides were highest in those sectors of society where individualism was the greatest and where social ties were most tenuous. The more integrated the society, the lower the suicide rates. Durkheim found higher percentages among Protestants over Catholics, among unmarried over married individuals, and among industrial workers. A strongly cohesive society restrains individuals from disposing of themselves because of the implicit taboo against suicide, and, more important, the sense of meaning such communities provide. The conclusion is inescapable: ethical individualism is ultimately self-destructive.

Another consequence of individualism is the loss of a sense of community. Interpersonal relationships become temporary and tentative, devoid of loyalty and commitment. Friendships are on the wane. Marriages become serial monogamy as the divorce rates continue to climb. Ethnic neighborhoods disappear, and housing tracts, with their collection of families, replace them. Where ethnic communities do exist, members often are embarrassed by their distinctives. By endorsing a "melting pot" approach to ethnic communities we have in fact destroyed distinctive communities for the sake of the homogeneity of a white middle-class community. Individualism, then, tends to destroy primary associations of friendship, marriage, neighborhood, and community.

Traditional communities assume the priority of the community over against that of the individual. It has been repeatedly documented that at least one way of describing the emergence of modern societies is the decline of traditional communities and the emergence of autonomous individuals. Mannheim (1936) and Homans (1974) have made the case that modern psychology as a discipline emerged from the dissolution of an unambiguously perceivable world order and the fragmentation of a stable worldview. Medieval society managed a consensus through its rituals and theology. The Reformation represented a breaking of this consensus by producing and legitimating a variety of worldviews. It shifted from an objective theology to a philosophy of the subject. Descartes made the doubting self the point of departure for epistemology. Following suit, Kant took the a priori categories of time and space contained in individual rationality as given for any theory of knowledge. The discipline of psychology emerged to give shape and form to the problem of structuring the needs of the isolated individual.

Individualism, Religion, and Psychology

Much of North American psychology has served to reinforce the individualistic view of the individual and to further the process of creating a society that values individualism (Gross, 1978; Hogan, 1975; Shur, 1976). Sarason (1974), in a most significant book, has criticized North American psychology for its commitment to individualism. Given the individualistic nature of American society, Albee (1977) concludes that American psychology has thus been made

> the most popular of all subjects. The glorification of self, the elevation of the peer group as the arbiter of reality, the rise of existential neurosis, and the hunger of the bleary eyed TV consumer for a new reality have sent all those people searching for meaning to the doorstep of the psychologist and the psychotherapist. Supply grows to meet demand. The preparation of persons aspiring to be psychotherapists seems all but out of control (1977:159).

In his study of individualism in American society, Robert Bellah and his associates (1985) interviewed a therapist they name Margaret Oldham. Her values include the importance of diversity in human experiences and the responsibility to be tolerant. For her to build and remain in community is too much like staying in the comfort of the womb rather than dealing with the reality of everyday life. Thus she finds herself able to get along much more easily with a greater variety of people than were her more moralistic parents. The most important thing in life, she says, is doing what one chooses to do as well as one can. Her hope is that individuals will accept responsibility for their own acts and communicate what they need and feel clearly. In therapy her hope is to enable individuals to achieve greater self-understanding and deal more realistically with life. The following is a transcript of a portion of the interview with Margaret regarding responsibility for another human being.

> Q: So what are you responsible for?
> A: I'm responsible for my acts and for what I do.
> Q: Does that mean you are responsible for others, too?
> A: No.
> Q: Are you your sister's keeper?
> A: No.
> Q: Your brother's keeper?
> A: No.
> Q: Are you responsible for your husband?
> A: I'm not. He makes his own decisions. He is his own person. He acts his own acts. I can agree with him or I can disagree with him. If I ever find him nauseous enough, I have a responsibility to leave and not deal with it anymore.

Q: What about children?
A: I . . . would say I have a legal responsibility for them, but in a sense they in turn are responsible for their own acts (1985:304).

Observations

When one focuses directly on the ways in which individualism has influenced the direction American psychology and psychotherapists have taken, the following observations can be made.

Sometimes psychologists and pastoral counselors have blatantly affirmed ethical individualism. Existentialist psychologists have repeatedly emphasized the uniqueness of the individual against a monolithic society that simply absorbs the person. To identify with social roles is to be self-deceived. Fritz Perls (1969) has maintained that "the richest person, the most productive creative person is a person who has no character. In our society we demand a person have a character, and especially a good character, because then you are predictable, and you can be pigeonholed, and so on" (14). Predictability is what society creates; uniqueness is what the individual naturally possesses.

The legitimate place for privacy is changed by some contemporary psychologists into an obsession with states of subjectivity (Back, 1978). Experiencing various and intense feelings is the goal of many advocates of personality development. One is encouraged to get in touch with one's feelings, to experience the extreme dualities of pain and joy, to risk spontaneity, and adjust to the flow of emotion. One is urged to express one's feelings rather than to conceal them. Primal scream therapy, EST, Gestalt therapy, all encouraged the same emphasis on subjectivity. Shur (1976) has complained that these approaches assume that

> somehow human beings can act and interact within a social and moral vacuum. That social structures and forms are meaningless and unnecessary. That unhappiness is due to our not realizing ourselves. That 'openness' and honesty will cause conflict and discontent to disappear. That learning certain content-free interpersonal skills will help ensure that we lead satisfying lives. That the very process of experiencing is more important than what it is that we experience (3).

What one experiences becomes the foundation of moral conduct. The contemporary individualist is one who can stand back objectively from all moral and cultural claims in order to criticize them. The emotivist self assumes cultural resources but, in fact, has no social identity nor a view of human life as order to a given end. The emotivist is one who cannot be unconditionally identified with any particular moral point of view. Ethical individualism is accepted in modernity and it is presumed that moral claims to objectivity and universality cannot be made good. MacIntyre (1981) comments that

> the specifically modern self, the self that I have called emotivist, finds no limits set to that on which it may pass judgment for such limits could only derive from rational criteria for evaluation, and as we have seen, the emotivist self lacks any such criteria. Everything may be criticized from whatever standpoint the self has adopted, including the self's choice of standpoint to adopt. It is in this capacity of the self to evade any necessary identification with any particular contingent state of affairs that some modern philosophers, both analytical and existentialist, have seen the essence of moral agency. To be a moral agent, on this view, is precisely to be able to stand back from any and every situation in which one is involved, from any and every characteristic that one may possess, and to pass judgment on it from a purely universal and abstract point of view that is totally detached from all social particularity. Anyone and everyone can thus be a moral agent, since it is in the self and not in social roles and practices that moral agency has to be located (1981:30).

In a most provocative book, Holifield (1983) has traced the transformation of Protestant pastoral counseling in America. Over the past four hundred years we have moved from "an ideal of otherworldly salvation to an implicit ethic of self-realization in American Protestantism" (1983:11). "The story proceeds from an ideal of self-denial to one of self-love, from self-culture to self-mastery to self-realization within a trustworthy culture, and finally to a later form of self-realization counterpoised against cultural mores and social institutions" (1983:12). He suggests that pastoral counseling has mirrored the changes in American religion, social and economic patterns, and the helping professions.

American pastoral care traditions are rooted in an ancient introspective piety which demands that Christian clergy possess a
knowledge of the inner world. It would not be outrageous to suggest that the extraordinary preoccupation with psychology in
twentieth century America owes something to the heritage of
experiential piety; that America became a nation of psychologists in part because it had been a land of Pietists (1983:65).

A similar point has been made by Hunter (1981, 1982)
regarding the privatization of evangelical culture. He has
delineated the ways in which evangelicalism has capitulated to
individualism. He argues that evangelicalism has responded to
the pluralism of modernity with increased subjectivization.
This has involved

an incessant preoccupation with the hitherto "undiscovered"
complexities of the self. Evangelicalism accommodates to this
cultural situation by expanding the parameters of its theodicy.
No longer does the conservative Protestant theodicy deal exclusively with the problems of suffering, grief, and death. Included
within the new theodicy are the attempts to cope with the end-
less musing of modern intra-subjectivity: "psychic balance,"
"emotional maturity," "self-actualization" and so on (1982:39).

**Most mental health professions and the religious com-
munity have developed models of the healthy individual
but they have been unable to articulate a positive vision
of the good community.** We have been preoccupied with
defining the healthy functioning of the individual. Thus we
focus primarily on harmony of internal states, personal actualization of goals, and individual freedom as the power to choose.
There is an emphasis on freedom from the shackles of oppressive parents, communities, and cultures. Self-fulfillment takes
precedence over community development. How individual
behavior contributes to the development of community tends
not to be specified. It has been naively assumed that if individuals are "healthy," a good community will be the natural consequence. One of the consequences of the absence of a vision of
the good society is that the psychologist or counselor cannot
invite the individual to some common ideal or standard of love,
marriage, or sacrifice.

Michael and Lisa Wallach (1983) state in their book, *Psychology's Sanction of Selfishness,* that psychologists have focused on motivation that occurs internally while remaining silent on motivation genuinely external to the self, even though such motivation may in fact prove therapeutic to the individual and the group. Psychologists have supported a preoccupation with self. The Wallachs suggest that individualism is especially apparent in social psychology texts where "social" is in quotes, where relationship to society is described in terms of conformity, and where self-sacrifice is limited to altruism. Helping others is reducing stress in one's self. They suggest that focus on psychological androgyny is, in fact, one more example of the importance of self-sufficiency and the irrelevance of others for self-completion. They point out that when psychologists do create a group context for growth, the express goal is still self-actualization rather than group actualization. One needs only to examine the nature of the group created. It meets for only a short period of time and then disbands. It has no history since members are thrown together as strangers. The group has no significant rituals beyond those that they possess as Westerners, and even then ritual is suspect.

The structure of therapy has placed the therapist and pastoral counselor between the individual and society, and it has been assumed that the healer will identify with the troubled individual. According to Phillip Rieff (1959, 1966), therapy that operates with an individualistic view of human nature and society will enable the individual to negotiate the transactions between biological urges, which are assumed given, and the excessive demands of the internalized cultural conscience. The therapist or counselor assumes a critical stance vis-à-vis community, and guards the patient against its negative effects. It is a therapy of release and remission, rather than one of confrontation and guilt based on social expectations.

The modern individualist seeks to preserve religious tradition but without personal and corporate discipline. Such an individual does not seek the connection between historical institutions and an interior worldview and too often pits human nature against the social order. The communication of ideals is under suspicion. It is the self that becomes the center as communities continue to disintegrate. This self seeks little beyond a manipulable sense of well-being. The psychological individual is a diplomat who negotiates with the moral demand system.

What are the implications for the therapist? The modern therapist, Rieff argues,

> speaks for the individual buried alive, as it were, in the culture. Thus to be freed from a tyrannical cultural super-ego is to be properly bedded in the present world. . . . The modern therapeutic idea is to empty those meanings that link the individual to dying worlds by assents of faith for which his analystic reason tells him he is not truly responsible. In this way, by acts of interpretation, the sacred becomes symptom. Sacred images are, then, the visible form, not of grace, but of sickness (1966:77).

This has meant that the substance of therapy is analystic in nature. The therapist provides interpretations of internal states, not external expectations of society. Therapy is not the mutual discovery of wisdom accumulated over millennia of human civilization, much less the return of the individual to meaningful communities. Such an approach to therapy only serves to undermine the validity of communal activity and to reinforce individualism.

Given the individualistic nature of North American society, therapeutic ethics are shaped more by the language of contract than relationship. In an individualistic society, relationships quickly degenerate into contractual relationships. In Western societies relationships have become oriented primarily to the market. However, if therapy is primarily a contractual relationship, the larger social context of therapeutic rituals is lost. Gone is the rich fabric of relationships and rituals in which the therapeutic ritual obtains its meaning, legitimation, and effectiveness. To the extent that therapy is isolated from vital communities with covenantal, sacrificial relationships, it becomes contractual and eventually ineffective.

The troubled individual is assumed to have all the moral resources necessary for healing to take place. Rogers (1961) assumes that each person possesses an innate capacity for growth and that the person's nature is essentially trustworthy: "I have little sympathy with the rather prevalent concept that man is basically irrational, and that his impulses, if not controlled, will lead to the destruction of others and self" (194).

Therapists tend to assume that in an individualistic society the troubled individual has the rational, emotional, and volitional resources necessary for healing. Hence the confused individual in therapy may be encouraged to take charge, to assume responsibility for personal conduct. It is assumed that the cognitive capabilities of the individual are adequate for understanding the nature of the personal problem. Or the individual is considered to possess the moral/ethical commitments necessary for change to occur.

But in an individualistic society, we are at a point where the emotionally confused individual brings few resources. Troubled individuals bring few compelling symbols, rituals, stories, traditions, practices, or authorities that they share in common with the therapist or counselor. But it is precisely to these resources that a therapist or counselor must appeal in order for healing to take place. Their absence insures the ineffectiveness of highly individualistic models of therapy.

Our techniques of healing have tended to reinforce ethical individualism by accepting as final moral authority either the therapist or the troubled individual. Given the fact that the therapeutic ritual is increasingly occurring in a moral vacuum, therapists or counselors tend to assume a stance of either objective neutrality or moralistic imperialism. In the first case the emotionally confused individual is seen as the final authority in ethical matters. To be directive is to make the troubled individual dependent rather than self-reliant. To be directive is to violate the sanctity of the individual right to self-determination. Thus, to counsel from clear and explicit values of health and well-being is to pass judgment on the emotionally confused individual for failing to live up to these moral ideals. We tend then to focus on acceptance, congruence, empathy, and forgiveness. There is no need to further the effects of an oppressive conscience. Rather, ego-controls need to be strengthened and overbearing guilt removed.

On the other hand there is the therapist or counselor who is clearly directive. Perhaps because the therapist or counselor assumes there is a consensus on the values in question, or because of the therapist's or counselor's own personality, it is assumed that being directive is acceptable. But that too is problematic because in an individualistic society there is no consensus of values and hence the position of the therapist is arbitrary. When consensus is absent, moralism is inevitable for the directive therapist. To base one's counsel entirely on personal experience is obviously individualistic.

The lifestyle of the therapist tends to reflect our individualistic society. Perhaps one of the most devastating effects of individualism is on the healer's personal life. The primary evidence for this is the loss of a sense of community. One's individual work is not seen in relation to a larger whole regardless of whether the issue is accountability, social responsibility, the importance of ritual, or the quality of legitimation. One's work is not tested against any tradition (beyond the professional one), nor is it expected that the lifestyle of the therapist or counselor reflect a positive community. When healers lose their sense of social responsibility, questions of injustice become secondary.

Furthermore, one's efforts are directed to troubled individuals first and foremost, not the creation of meaningful communities, traditions, rituals, and symbols. The development of a world of shared meanings is assumed to occur in the context of dyadic relationships: therapist and troubled individual.

Lastly, legitimation is assumed to have occurred with licensure. But the legitimation of a narcissistic community only perpetuates the disease. A critical question then is: which community or culture legitimates and sanctions the therapeutic event?

The view of religion assumed by psychologists and pastoral counselors has tended to be individualistic. Lawrence Kohlberg's (1968) theory of moral development is consistent with the liberal view of individual autonomy. I will examine this theory later in greater detail. Moral development begins with the stage in which the child's behavior is dominated by institutional control of consequences. The child then passes through a stage where morality is mere convention or social custom, and emerges later as a mature moral individual who can decide moral-ethical dilemmas on the basis of the rational use of moral principles, and act accordingly. The cognitive transformations prerequisite to moral development are given through natural interaction between the child and the environment. A normative community makes no significant contribution to the shape of this process of development.

The argument here is not so much to demonstrate that all of contemporary psychology is imbued with individualism. There are many notable exceptions. But there is nevertheless a strong individualistic element in our culture. At the Harvard commencement exercises in 1978, Alexander Solzhenitsyn roundly criticized the West for its lack of courage and moral fiber. The root of the problem, he said, was to be found in the West's uncritical acceptance of Enlightenment individualism, the autonomy of the person from cultural and moral constraints. The inevitable result, said Solzhenitsyn, is the decline of spirituality. The material success of the West has precluded the suffering prerequisite for moral and cultural development.

There is a cancer destroying the body politic of Western societies. That cancer is the idolatrous worship of the individual. What was once a benign concern for the emancipation of the person from oppressive traditions has now become a malignancy that threatens the destruction of tradition and community itself. The pervasiveness of this cancer is evident in the loss of such vital signs as the ability to voluntarily sacrifice personal interests for the sake of the other and the willingness to be held accountable for one's actions. The quality of therapy and our congregational life is fundamentally contingent upon the extirpation of this cancer and the development of alternatives.

5

Signposts along the Way

The L'Arche communities for the developmentally disabled were begun by Jean Vanier (1981, 1989), a Catholic, a philosopher, and a deeply caring person. In the early sixties, after teaching philosophy at the University of Toronto for several years, Vanier left for France. His bishop suggested he consider inviting two retarded adults to live with him. After 20 years, they still have not parted. In fact, some fifty communities with the disabled have sprung up around the world in response to that act of caring. The basis of the L'Arche communities is an ethical commitment to the rejected.

The power of a true story lies in its ability to create a people whose lives reflect that story. In their charter, the L'Arche communities state that their first aim is "to create communities inspired by the Beatitudes and the Spirit of the Gospel." Some years ago I visited three L'Arche communities in Canada. I was deeply moved by their communal life. L'Arche is a community of healing, not an institution. There is always a balance between the number of disabled and nondisabled participants in the community so as to avoid the pitfalls of institutionalization. It is not primarily a place of work, though work is done; it is where the helpers live with the disabled. It is a place to come to serve the disabled and receive the gift they have to give us. By participating in their suffering, assistants experience Christ's presence and thus grow personally.

The celebration around meals and work is exuberant. Work is important in the development of this sense of community. It is assumed that work has dignity. All are expected to participate according to their ability in the necessary tasks of community maintenance. The spirit of capitalism is absent since the goal of the community is not efficiency and high productivity, but the cultivating of gifts, and being a faithful presence to the disabled. Such a community is not a restriction of freedom for the disabled but an expansion of it. For the assistants it is voluntary sacrifice.

Though a human community fraught with the frailties of all humanity, in many ways the L'Arche community illustrates the vision articulated in the first section on the role of the Reign of God. There is an overarching Christian worldview and a compelling ethic. Individualism is rejected and individuality is affirmed. There is a clear commitment to liberation and accessibility to the poor. It is a sign of the coming Reign of God. The L'Arche communities point to a clear consensus among them about the nature of their calling, the nature of their community, and the nature of their responsibility to the disabled. There is a sense of mission that emerges out of a covenant with God and with one another. The division between the disabled and the able is broken down—and that in itself is no small sign of the presence of the Reign of God.

In this chapter I will make the case that we desperately need a renewed sense of community and that it is in the quality of life of the Christian community that the content of moral language in therapy is illustrated and legitimated. The covenantal nature of Christian relationships becomes the model for the healing event (Yoder, 1972). If the church seeks to incarnate the story of the Reign of God, it must then see itself as a community that develops a coherent worldview consistent with this story. My objective is to make a case for the church as a primary community of ethical discernment for the professional therapist who seeks first the Reign of God. The church is called to develop a consensus not only on values and belief, but also in practice. When this is the case, then the Christian will be able to find a primary identity and locus of accountability in the concrete Christian community. The church as an ethical community is called to reflect the Reign of God historically. It is called to ethical reflection on the nature of its witness in the modern world. Ethical reflection in the context of the discerning church community is the foundation of its witness to society. The church is not only a place of worship, evangelism, and service, it is also a place where the people who confess Christ as Lord engage in a dialogue for consensus about the nature of their life together.

The Case for Community

Our views of personal identity, morality, therapy, and education are radically altered if we accept a communal perspective. In fact, it can be argued that to function at all requires an extant community. But before we examine the implications of a communal perspective for ethics and therapy, the notion of community needs more careful analysis. In the wake of the decline of liberalism, there is a reemergence of those seeing the importance of community.

In his book, *The Quest for Community,* Robert Nisbet (1953) provides us with this excellent summary of the meaning of community:

> By community I mean something that goes far beyond mere local community. The word, as we find it in much nineteenth- and twentieth-century thought encompasses all forms of relationship which are characterized by a high degree of personal intimacy, emotional depth, moral commitment, social cohesion, and continuity in time. Community is founded on man conceived in his wholeness rather than in one or another of the roles, taken separately, that he may hold in a social order. It draws its psychological strength from levels of motivation deeper than those of mere volition or interest, and it achieves its fulfillment in a submergence of individual will that is not possible in unions of mere convenience or rational assent. Community is a fusion of feeling and thought, of tradition and commitment, of membership and volition. It may be found in, or be given symbolic expression by, locality, religion, nation, race, occupation, or crusade. Its archetype, both historically and symbolically, is the family, and in almost every type of genuine community the nomenclature of family is prominent. Fundamental to the strength of the bond of community is the real or imagined antithesis formed in the same social setting by the noncommu-

nal relations of competition or conflict, utility or contractual
assent. These, by their relative impersonality and anonymity,
highlight the close personal ties of community (1953:47–48).

A community then, provides a home (Buber, 1965) for the person. It assumes that personal fulfillment is a consequence of a
community with an integrated symbol system, a vision of an
ideal character, the encouragement necessary for discipline,
and the mercy appropriate for failure. The survivability of the
community depends, among other things, on the quality of
individual commitment to its purposes.

Symbolic interactionists have sought to articulate a community perspective (Mead, 1934). They emphasize the place of ritual, social roles, and institutions to provide a stable context in
which the individual can function. Beliefs that give meaning
and direction to personal pilgrimages emerge out of the history
of experiences of a particular people (Berger and Luckman,
1966). At its best the values of the community are implicitly
accepted and shape behavior. Relationships between individuals are bound by covenants and a sense of interdependency.
Identity is then a function of knowing one's place in the community and accepting its history as one's own. The expectation
that the self must have limits is accepted for the sake of harmony in the community.

Community, Church, and the Individual

From the perspective of community the liberal dimensions
of individuality listed in the previous chapter would be interpreted as follows: 1) The diversity of abilities and personalities
in a community are affirmed and uniqueness is seen as flour-
ishing in a supportive environment. A sense of uniqueness is a
function also of the larger sense of corporate uniqueness of
vision. 2) Autonomy of reason and choice are assumed to be
critical for the development of quality of life in the community,
but autonomy is not to displace accountability, which is shaped
by the collective wisdom of many generations. Every community also needs its critics if it is to grow, but if it is composed
of only prophets it will not survive. 3) Privacy is the locus of
personal discipline. By nature, however, we are social, interde-
pendent. Hence, we cannot dichotomize public and private

except in abstraction from life. 4) Self-development is recognized as important, but not exclusive of cultural development, lest one deplete the reservoir of resources of a community. Personal growth may well emerge indirectly out of service to the cultural whole. 5) An emphasis on culture and community does not violate the sanctity of the individual. If community becomes an end in itself, then we have the same horror that is produced when the individual becomes an end.

The Five Dimensions of Individuality

From the perspective of Christianity as community and the church as community, the five dimensions of individuality discussed above are further interpreted below.

Uniqueness

In the context of the Christian community, the uniqueness of the individual is not lost. Just as the personal relationship of the individual is not absorbed into the divine as some mystics might assume, so also the individual is not dissolved in the Christian community. The apostle Paul wrote: "Now you are the body of Christ and individually members of it" (1 Cor. 12:27). Uniqueness is affirmed in terms of the diversity of gifts that individual members possess. These gifts are not distributed in the people of God according to class, sex, age, or formal education; nor is uniqueness sacrificed to social position or stereotype. Jesus' relationships with women, the poor, or Samaritans are reminders that the indeterminate quality of the individual must never be substituted with classifications or categories.

However, nowhere in the story of the Hebrews or the early Christians is uniqueness an end in itself. Diversity is not valued apart from unity. The uniqueness of the individual's experiences, abilities, and skills are not so much sacrificed at the altar of the community as they are first corporately discerned, recognized, nurtured, and used in the service of the church in the world. When the diversity of unique individuals is made absolute, then the unity of any community, including the church, is jeopardized. Common unity is a theme that is repeatedly emphasized in the Scriptures. Jesus prays for the disciples that their small community might manifest a unity that reflects his own relationship with the Father (John

17:22–23). Paul is similarly concerned about the Roman church (Rom. 14:1–15, 18), the Corinthian church (1 Cor. 1–5), and the Philippian church (Phil. 2:2). Such unity is not uniformity of thought or even of practice.

Independence

While a qualified sense of independence contributes to community, unbridled autonomy is blatantly destructive. In fact, in the Judeo-Christian tradition autonomy is viewed as one of the root causes of alienation from self, others, and God. Humanity seeks to be freed from the will of God for ordered human life. Obedience and autonomy are incongruent (Brueggeman, 1979).

Independence of the individual is understood within the context of a covenant relationship with Yahweh and a covenant with a people (Brueggeman, 1979). That covenant is entered voluntarily and carries obligations (Exod. 24; Josh. 24). Commitment to the covenant means loyalty to that binding relationship. The criteria by which the quality of the covenant is measured are faithfulness, obedience, and justice. Law emerges from the covenant relationship. The law was the external manifestation of the covenant. In the mind of a Hebrew the law was never synonymous with moralism (Toews, 1982). The Psalmist could say, "Oh, how I love your law" (Ps. 119:97). In the New Testament, God has made a covenant of love, forgiveness, and faithfulness through Jesus Christ. The church community is a consequence of the common covenant with God. The expression of that covenant in the life of the individual Christian is a life of discipleship and obedience to Jesus Christ.

From the nature of the covenant relationship with Yahweh and with fellow members in the covenant, one derives accountability to God in the midst of a people. To be accountable means to give account. It is important for the sake of relationships to interpret our actions to our brothers/sisters (Gish, 1979). This may mean being accountable to a specific person, to a small group of believers, or to my fellow believers in Nigeria. Independence and individuality need not militate against openness to correction in the life of the Church. In the New Testament community it was expected that Christians respond to the erring member (Matt. 18:15–18). The church community is then a community of moral discernment. It has been given the mandate to discern the spirits (1 Thess. 5:21), and what is good and acceptable and perfect (Rom. 12:2). It is not simply a matter of making up one's mind independent of the church but in concert with it. This is the context for the Christian for testing the leading of the Holy Spirit in our professions. Covenant making then implies openness to correction (Eph. 5:21) and the willingness to submit personal decisions to corporate examination. It is just as inconsistent to say that one is willing to submit to God and not to take into account the wisdom of brothers and sisters as it is to say that one loves God and then hates a brother. The covenant community is a community of moral discernment that provides a normative context for our life and work.

The focus on autonomy in the Enlightenment was to provide a place for prophetic dissent. However, for even the most radical of Old Testament prophets, the message was to return to faithful obedience, to covenant life in the midst of a covenanting community. Never is dissent viewed apart from covenant. Nor did the focus on covenant preclude freedom of choice. The covenant-making God is precisely the God who liberates from the bondage of Egypt. The covenant is freely entered and broken. Coercion is anathema. The basis of accountability is the freedom of entering a specific covenant agreement.

Privacy

The emphasis on personal privacy began as a corrective to intrusive institutions, but it degenerated in the twentieth century into an obsession with the subjective. It assumes a dichotomy of self and society. In contrast to this separation, the biblical story assumes the essentially social nature of humanity. Eve is created when God says that it is not good for a man to be alone. Karl Barth (1960) has made the point that the image of God in us is lodged in the possibility of relationship—male and female. The natural place in Hebrew society for the individual is in a harmonious relationship—shalom (Robinson, 1980; Wolff, 1974). It is the leper who dwells alone. When Hosea describes the misery of his people, he calls them "a wild ass alone by himself" (Hos. 8:9). Personal sin renders one unable to live peaceably with others. And when Yahweh does call one person—Abraham—to leave others behind, it is with a blessing that from him will proceed a great people—similar to the case of the individual prophet who experienced profound isolation. While prophets experience loneliness as they speak for Yahweh, they also invite their hearers to a new community. Thus individuality is conceived of in the context of corporateness in the biblical story. If one suffers, all suffer (1 Cor. 12:26); and the life of one affects all as leaven affects the whole loaf (1 Cor. 5:6). One person's gain is everyone's gain.

The notion of the communal nature of the personhood leads to the next step, which characterizes the relationships within the church community as openness, intimacy, and dialogue. Love is the glue that gives coherence to community. It makes free and open dialogue possible. It results in trust in others and the freedom to share deeply. Sharing one's innermost feelings is not an end in itself but occurs in the context of a committed community and for the purpose of both personal and corporate growth. It is sharing that continues over a period longer than a weekend encounter. Moreover, sharing implies the willingness to carry the burdens of others. Love included the willingness to share "private" property.

Self-Development

The development of the individual is certainly a concern of the Judeo-Christian tradition. However, in contrast to the pursuit of self-actualization, self-realization, and self-fulfillment, Jesus assumed that personal development comes only through self-sacrifice, dedication to the calling of reconciliation, and "building up" of the people of God. The submission to the will of God in the covenant finds expression in voluntary submission to the needs of others. Community cannot emerge unless there is sacrifice of self (O'Connor, 1976). The result is not self-deprecation, loss of integrity, or the creation of dependency. This is not passive surrender to a nebulous being or the status quo. Rather, self-affirmation, personhood, and wholeness are a result of sacrifice of self (Luke 14:33). Paul actually suggests that personal integrity may not always be as important as the needs of a fellow Christian (Stendahl, 1976). To order one's life by the weaker person is the example of love rather than integrity and the basis of the creating of community.

Moreover, in contrast to an obsession with personal enrichment, the New Testament is constantly calling the Christian to be involved in the building up of the life of the church. That occurs in ways already described above but also in the participation in the significant rituals of the church community: baptism, communion, infant dedication, marriages, funerals, etc. The quality of church life is a function of the quality of the activities it performs together: worship, service, work, study, play, and meals.

Sanctity of Life

While the sanctity and worth of the individual are recognized, the individual life is not seen as an end in itself, for that would preclude the legitimacy of martyrdom. Furthermore, the Christian tradition has at different times placed value on the importance of both the individual and the church. As a sign of the Reign of God, the church is God's agent of reconciliation in the world. The people of God are to be the moving force in history and are to give meaning and direction to it. In the Exodus event we have the paradigmatic event for an understanding of Yahweh as the people-creating God. The Israelites emerge as a people as a result of a covenant with the one true God who is the creator of both the human race and of the Jewish community. In direct continuity with the Old Testament story of the people of God, Jesus calls for the creation of a new people. He calls for the inauguration of the Reign of God. One immediate consequence is the emergence of the disciple community. It is community that is to be characterized by humility, reconciliation, a thirst for justice, and love. The church is an extension of this disciple community.

The Church and the "Rule of Christ"

Between the first and the twentieth centuries, a radical shift has taken place in the nature of our view of religious community. Once the church was a community marked by concern about its character; today we worry about worship style and church growth. Without rejecting these concerns, I wish to make a case for the old. The Reign of God, as Jesus described it, is a community of persons who have responded to the call to reflect the image of God. The New Testament church emerged in response to God's call to new personal and corporate life. The early Christians were recognized by their love one for the other, and their life together reflected a commitment to each other. The New Testament call for a people of God is an extension of the call to be a righteous people in the Old Testament. This community is governed by the "rule of Christ." The Sermon on the Mount is its charter. The example of Christ is its guide (Borg, 1988).

Recent New Testament scholarship has paid particular attention to first century Judaism in understanding the message of Jesus (Sanders, 1985). The discussion centers around the role of "law" in the New Testament community. If one takes seriously the role of law, then the perspective of the Christian community as a community of ethical conversation and praxis is reinforced. In the past, discussions of law in the New Testament were dominated by a paradigm that suggests that the law was abrogated or ended in Jesus, or it was so completely equated with love that it held no meaning. In his book *Jesus and Judaism,* E. P. Sanders (1985) explores the coherence between what Jesus had in mind, how he viewed his own relationship to his nation and his people's religion, the reason for his death, and the beginning of the Christian movement. Sanders's method is to search for the historical Jesus and to evaluate him in the light of the Gospels and in the context of first-century Palestine. The following picture emerges from the research.

Jesus Accepts the Law

Sanders argues that if the Synoptic Gospels are properly interpreted, there is no evidence to suggest that Jesus opposed the law. Issues of divorce, the Sabbath, food and cleanliness, and the passages relevant to these observances need not be interpreted to mean that Jesus overruled the law. What is crucial, according to Sanders, is that belief did not remove the law as the present mediator of God's will.

Jesus Fulfills the Law

Sanders posits that Jesus brings the law to fulfillment, that he did not step outside the boundaries of first-century Palestinian law theology. The law remains valid for teaching and obedience. Jesus affirms the validity of the law (Matt. 5:17–20). In his life he fulfills the law, specifically in his relationship to the poor. The essence of the law Jesus defines as love (Matt. 12:28–34; Mark 10:17–31). In fact, Jesus intensifies the demand of the law (Matt. 5:21–47). The concern of the law is to create the shape of God's people in the world. Jesus encourages the disciple community to engage in ethical discernment ("binding and loosing").

Jesus Is Both the Form and the Content of the Law

Barth (1959) argues that the law is the necessary form of the Gospel, while its content is grace. Barth immediately ties grace to the incarnation of Jesus Christ. Grace is not only acceptance. It is the fact that Jesus in his humanity stands with us in our humanity. But Jesus is also the law in that he fulfilled the law through imaginative obedience in his own life. If the law is the manifest will of God, then we see it made concrete at Bethlehem, Tiberias, Gethsemane, Golgotha, and on the road to Emmaus. When the will of God is done in Jesus the law is manifested to us. Grace is made concrete. When the word of grace is spoken, it makes a claim on our lives.

The work of the apostle Paul is an expansion of this new community in that he seeks to bring about reconciliation between Jew and Gentile (Stendahl, 1976). The new humanity, called the church, transcends race, social class, and sex (Gal. 3:18). The church is a sign of the Reign of God when it approximates this New Testament vision. W. D. Davies (1958) has argued that Paul must be seen as a Jew who observed the law all his life. Paul assumed the law was good, holy, just, and spiritual (Rom. 7). The purpose of the law was to reveal not only sin, but also the righteousness of Christ. For Paul, the law is fulfilled in Christ and is therefore to be observed as the new Messianic Torah. Davies pointed out that Paul deals with the law in the context of the Jew-Gentile relationship. Christ fulfills the law for the Jew by doing it, and for the Gentile by making possible their adoption into the promises of Abraham. Paul's theology of law is rooted in God's covenant with Israel. Paul makes the case that there need be no conflict between Jew and Greek because in Jesus Christ they are one. Jews do not need to become Gentiles, nor do Gentiles become Jews through observance of the law.

John Toews (1982) makes the case that for Paul the law is good. It is the gift of God (Rom. 7:7ff). Christ fulfilled the law for both Jew and Gentile (Rom. 3, 4; Gal. 3). Salvation comes by faith: both the faithfulness of God and the faith of believers, (Rom. 3:21ff). The law can be obeyed, but the power of sin prevents us (Rom. 9:30ff; Rom. 7:7). For Paul, the law judges human sin (Rom. 2, 5) and the law is fulfilled by love (Rom. 13). The fulfillment of the law is possible through the Holy Spirit and in the context of the church (Gal. 5; Rom. 8). To summarize, the church as a sign of the Reign of God is one that governs its life by the ethic of Jesus. The law (read "rule of Christ") is not odious, it is liberating. With a recovery of the goodness of law, then the Christian community can be a community of ethical conversation and praxis.

The Church as Ethical Community

From a point where the individual was accepted as God's unique creation, as God's covenant partner, and as member of God's family, Western Christendom has moved to a point where the individual stands alone before God. From the perspective of individualism, an emphasis on the organic nature of the church becomes incomprehensible. For those who do not identify with the church as the common center of faith, the uniqueness of the individual is seen as violated by a church that demands conformity and hence creates sheep. A common covenant among members is perceived as undermining independence and stifling creativity. Accountability for one's action to the larger church community is regarded as meddling. For those with this perspective the church becomes instead a support group for me "to do my own thing." Emphasis on the church as community is seen as institutional arrogance and the end of the dignity of the individual.

Given our analysis of culture in the previous section, the church is called to be a community with a distinctive worldview, compelling ethos, and a powerful story. But a Christian community does not spring up full blown. It emerges from small companies of committed persons who seek to be a reflection and sign of the presence of the Reign of God. The Christian story invites us to live the Christian life with others. Christianity is more than a conversion experience or an intense relationship with God. It is lived out in just relationships. It is a call to recognize no other god and tolerate no broken relationships. Ideally, Christians are a people who serve one another, forgive one another, love one another, encourage one another, and correct one another. I suggest that if we hope for the church to be a healing community, it must become a primary community, create a coherent praxis, and develop structures of accountability.

Primary Community

If the church is to be a community of ethical discernment it must become a *primary* community. The church will not be a community of ethical accountability if we accept ethical individualism. Either the client or the therapist can assume a position of an entirely independent ethical agent. Such individualism is inimical to a therapeutic process that reflects Christian values and churchly discernment. If an individualist ethical perspective is applied to the therapeutic profession, a number of questions are usually raised.

First, it might be argued that the therapist should not be considered an ethicist. His or her task is to focus on conflicted feelings, lack of communication, early traumas, cognitive aberrations, and interpersonal conflicts. These are not perceived as ethical issues. They are simply problems to be solved.

Second, it might be argued that the therapist is an ethicist, but accountable first and foremost to his or her own religious/ethical convictions. Those convictions are seen as shaped not by a communal process but by individual experience. It is the individual healer who defines the substance of moral language.

Third, it might be argued that the client is the final authority in ethical matters that emerge in healing. After all, respect for the client demands that one begin where the client is. In this argument the client is no more accountable to a moral community than is the therapist. To talk then of healing as a moral affair leads inevitably to the charge of moralism and imposition.

We submit that all three of these positions subvert the church as a community that provides an ethical context for the healer and the healing process. We assume that many of the ethical issues that the healer encounters are issues that the church too is called to be concerned about: the nature of individual freedom, abortion, sexual and verbal abuse, loss of personal dignity, economics and social class, use of private or research information, discrimination, etc.

It is my fundamental understanding that the therapist in the Christian community is an ethicist—i.e., one who engages in discerning behavior appropriate to the establishment of the Reign of God. Moreover, while the individual healer can engage in ethical discernment apart from an ethical community, the church as a community needs the therapist as a significant member of the discernment process. The values of the Reign of God guide the process of discernment of the church and the Christian therapist. Church and world are not ontologically different. Rather, the difference is in the nature of their confessions. One confesses that Jesus is Lord, the other does not. It is the exploration of this conviction that makes the church a community of discernment. It is the church that is called to make the Reign of God visible (Col. 3:12–17). The first responsibility of the church is to *be* the church. The church does not *have* a social ethic, it *is* a social ethic. It is the place where the stories of Jesus are told and enacted.

To be sure, Christ's presence is not confined to the church since the Reign of God extends beyond the church, but it is in the context of the church that our ethical convictions are to be formed. The normative context for discernment for Christians is the community of people who self-consciously and self-critically covenant with God and each other to live a life consistent with the Christian story. The story and the discernment of its implications are normative in relationship to all other traditions. The church must set its own agenda in the midst of the world. In so doing, the church may in fact help modernity to understand that morality is fragmented, abstract, and individualistic, and that we have few resources for healing. For that practical reason, it is imperative that the church be a primary community for Christians.

Common Praxis

If the church is to be a community of discernment, it must develop a *common praxis*. Therapy is not simply an individual affair. The Christian who counsels is dependent on the nature and quality of the Christian community. Good counsel is dependent on communal life that is justly lived, love that is freely given, and service that is joyfully rendered. When the Christian community is unfaithful there will be fewer resources available for healing that are consistent with the vision of the Reign of God. It takes a righteous community to nurture the compelling ethic necessary for healing.

The church is called to discern the will of God in its historical setting. The New Testament church certainly did when it convened a meeting in Jerusalem to discuss the role of the Gentiles in the life of the church (Acts 15). Paul's letters to the churches are replete with advice and concern about the ethical quality of their life. The unity for which Christ prays is not simply one of attitude but one of consistent discipleship (John 17). Thus, the community of faith is a community of praxis.

The power of a moral language to create change in therapy is related to the existence of real communities that incarnate that language in history. To talk of love for the poor makes sense and is compelling because there are communities such as L'Arche that have done it. One wonders what occurs in the therapeutic rituals of Christian healers when their religious communities fail to engage in the casuistry necessary to give material content to the moral language necessary for healing. The temptation will be to arbitrarily assign such meanings oneself, simply allow the client to do so, or to accept the prevailing cultural ethic.

What we need is a commitment to ethical discernment and dialogue by the church. Hauerwas (1981) states:

> What I mean by casuistry, is not just the attempt to adjudicate difficult cases of conscience within a system of moral principles, but it is the process by which a tradition tests whether its practices are consistent (that is, truthful) or inconsistent in the light of its basic habits and convictions or whether these convictions require new practices and behavior (1981:120).

The church, as a community of conviction, seeks to provide content to its moral language. For example, such terms as freedom, assertiveness, and equality are abstract and have little material content.

The church as a community of moral discourse gives meaning to its ethical terms. To use such terms as freedom and equality as values that are Christian and hence appropriate in a theory of government or therapy neglects the fact that these terms have material content in Jesus' definition of the Kingdom and as they are incarnated in His life and death. Ethical terms are not self interpreting but require a tradition to give them content (1981:134).

Our moral language must be compared with the Sermon on the Mount and Jesus's definition of God's Reign as it is incarnated in his life and death.

Groome (1980) also sees the church as a community of shared praxis. He rejects a dichotomy between theory and practice in favor of a dialectic between reflection and action. By a shared praxis Groome means "a group of Christians sharing in dialogue their critical reflection on present action in light of the Christian story and its vision toward the end of lived Christian faith" (1980:184). He suggests five components of a shared praxis. The first is actual present action or engagement in the world. Second, critical reflection calls one to evaluate the present, to uncover the past in the present, and to envision the future in the present. On the one hand it critiques ideology and on the other it creatively imagines the future. The third component is dialogue. It is a conversation in which individual stories are shared and disclosed. The fourth component is the Christian story as we find it in the whole faith tradition and expressed or embodied in a people. Our story is that God has acted in history and our call is to conform our actions to that history. The last stage is the vision that emerges from the story. Here we strategize how one lives the story in the midst of history. Groome suggests three ways that our praxis can be tested. Are the consequences consistent with making the Reign of God present (Matt. 7:20)? Is there continuity with the Christian story? Is the substance of our praxis consistent with the teaching of the church?

Structures of Accountability

If the church is to be a visible sign of the Reign of God, then it must develop *structures of accountability* for its members. Too often the church has assumed that the nature and quality of its life is such that it is *already* an ethical community. The "three plus ten" model—i.e., Sunday morning, Sunday night, Wednesday evening, plus ten percent tithe—is simply not enough to create a community of ethical discourse. Very few resources are built up with such a meager commitment to the righteous life of the church. The ethical individualism of Western societies is apparent also in the church. When that is the case, there is little commitment to ethical conversation. Hence the church's responsibility, if it wishes to be an ethical community, is to attend to the quality of its own life.

Farnsworth (1985) has called for an embodied integration that extends beyond the intellectual to an integration of theory and practice. Practically, Farnsworth suggests that establishing a reference group of believers would be an example of bringing one's counseling under the Lordship of Christ and being professionally accountable. The group would be composed of professional and lay individuals. Here one would have a forum for discussion of one's counseling goals, frustrations, dilemmas, and hopes.

The L'Arche community serves as a model. First, it is a community in which religious ideology shapes the ethos. Such a community emerges as a result of careful reflection on the nature of the Christian story as normative for healing. While it is a community of comfort to the disabled, it is also a community that has carefully discerned its calling and how it will help. It is an ethical community that seeks, in creative ways, to be accessible to the poor and devalued in society. Also, the assistants view themselves as extensions of the community and as instruments of its vision. The L'Arche community is then a healing resource because it has discerned the implications of its story for the healing event and has incorporated those convictions in its own life. In so doing it has provided us with some ethical guidelines for the healing process, created an alternative context for healing, and infused culture with a healing story.

Conclusion

A community that emerges because its members have a common vision, a commitment to voluntary sacrifice of personal interests for the sake of the other person, and has a common language with which and through which it describes what it values and what is the nature of the world, is easily perceived as demanding conformity by an individualist culture. Communally developed convictions are perceived as fixed legalisms. The separation from other communities that is a natural consequence of a particular vision, set of commitments, and network of beliefs is viewed as provincialism and sectarianism. The desire to maintain continuity with the past generations of believers is rejected as traditionalism. The order and predictability that develop naturally over time in any community is perceived by the disenchanted as an overprotective, secure environment that requires no risks and is suspicious of novelty and variety.

However, if the problem endemic to individualism is social amnesia, the temptation inherent in an emphasis on community and tradition is authoritarianism, conservatism, and positivism. The first sacrifices the individual to the collectivity and, hence, fuels the objections of liberalism. Conservatism in its worst form rejects experimentation, innovation, variety, and creativity. Positivism simply accepts the structure of a particular social organization as given and assumes that the individual must be socialized into its ideals. The question then is one of knowing how to evaluate a given society and constructing an alternative vision.

What is most troubling is the incredible disarray of the very community that is to serve as a model and context of our healing and to which we are accountable. I speak of the church. I may encourage therapists to take the church seriously only to find that the church itself will not take ethical discernment seriously. The healing professions are not alone in experiencing the devastating effects of individualism. The church too has felt its impact. Some would say the church has become a collection of individuals. The Lord's Supper is taken in serial fashion. Rituals of healing are not really effective. Fellowship is eating together, not sharing our visions and frustrations. The life of the church becomes simply a base for me to do my own thing. When we assume that religious experience is synonymous with individual experience, a personal relationship to God, there is little concern about the quality of relationships. There is then no clear consensus about what behaviors we are willing to call Christian. We appear to be more concerned about the salvation of individuals than we are about ethical discernment. Gone is any hard wrestling with questions that face professionals working in our culture. To talk of covenant making is threatening. To hold an individual accountable is meddling. When individualism overtakes the church there is fundamentally no center that holds the church together. What little community there remains in the life of the church is perceived as demanding conformity. What behavioral expectations it develops are seen as legalistic. It stifles creativity and destroys uniqueness. If the professions are in trouble, so is the church.

The Christian professional has then two responsibilities: to *help* the Church to *be* the Church, and to counsel with the Reign of God as context. The question that we face is our own responsibility to develop creative models of the Church and compelling Christian symbols in the twentieth century. That will come with both a cosmic vision of the Reign of God and the awareness of the Church as a mustard seed, a small sign of that coming reign.

Just as individualism is a deterrent to the development of community and an understanding of the church as an ethical community, so also there is competition once the church is considered a significant social entity. Professions provide another context in which to make our work meaningful. They are alternate ethical communities. The issue is not whether we must choose between them but how we negotiate a relationship in which each is nurtured. That is the focus of the next chapter. The final chapter in this section will explore five strategies the church has used throughout history to interact with the larger world of culture. The relationship of these strategies to the field of psychology will also be explored.

Professional:
To Be or Not to Be?

The professions are repeatedly the object of a barrage of criticisms. Our age has been characterized (Illich, 1977) as "the age of disabling professions." In such an era the experts have taken control, adjudicated needs, nurtured dependence, and sapped resources. Professionals, so the argument proceeds, have socialized the uninitiated into the dominant values of the cultural elite they represent. By virtue of their institutionalized power, a presumably esoteric body of knowledge, and a specialized language, the professional emerges as the new high priest who decides who shall be healed, when, and for how much. A new population (and market) of people springs up with the label of "clients." Meanwhile lay persons have lost their ability to think and do for themselves.

Currently the critique of the professions revolves around their ability to monitor their members. To what extent do members of the profession reflect the ethical code? Specifically, are they competent to render the services they advertise, are clients sexually harassed, is there price gouging, etc.? That which ought to occupy the most time of professional organizations—namely, monitoring its members through peer review mechanisms—is largely lacking. At least part of the present tension with managed care is the fact that mental health professionals have not developed their own peer review organizations. Mental health practitioners have operated like independent entrepreneurs. There is a widespread criticism of utilization review. If the reviewer is one who lacks the training to evaluate a case, objections are understandable. But to reject all utilization review on the grounds that it is an invasion of privacy could, in fact, be an evasion of accountability. Supervision is part of training. Why not assume it is a part of professional growth?

Healing rituals in Western societies are extremely private. That also makes accountability to external communities difficult. The Christian community has little idea whether the therapeutic relationship is sexist, whether the resources of God's story are utilized, or whether the ethical position of the church on abortion, divorce, sexual faithfulness (for example), is considered. As a member of the Christian community, the individual therapist is a representative of its story. Therapy, then, is never simply a private practice. The individual therapist is responsible to demonstrate that what transpires in the therapeutic process is consistent with the Christian story. The church is responsible for developing a moral vocabulary appropriate to our social existence, and to incarnate its convictions in its daily life.

In this chapter I wish to explore the relationship between two social structures: the Christian community and the mental health professions (see Good and Kraybill, 1982). At the outset I submit that the process of professionalization can serve as a significant contributor to the effectiveness of the therapist; it can also neutralize the critical edge of our witness. However, unless we are self-critical, professional communities and the church tend both to reflect and reinforce the values of society. To the extent that a Christian professional senses a call to be a part of God's people, to that extent professionalization must at least be qualified, but not necessarily rejected. It is our task to select the best of the professional tradition in the service of the Reign of God. That, I submit, is the responsibility of both the Christian community and the professional.

The Profession as Ethical Community

Professional communities are not simply loose associations that provide its members with news and liability insurance. I wish to argue that professional communities are ethical communities on the same order as religious communities. They expect a measure of loyalty, demand conformity on critical standards, and often reflect society's most treasured values. In what follows I will explore what it means to say that profession is a community and, more specifically, an ethical community.

First, what is meant by being "professional"? Together with William Goode (1957), I would maintain that an essential dimension of established and aspiring professions is a sense of community. He lists the following as characteristics of the community:

1. Its members are bound by a sense of identity.
2. Once in it, few leave, so that it has a continuing status for the most part.
3. Its members share values in common.
4. Its role definitions vis-à-vis both members and non-members are agreed upon and are the same for all members.
5. Within the areas of communal action there is a common language, which is understood only partially by outsiders.
6. The community has power over its members.
7. Its limits are reasonably clear, though they are not physical and geographical, but social.
8. Though it does not produce the next generation biologically, it does so socially through its control over the selection of professional trainees, and through its training processes it sends these recruits through an adult socialization process (Good, 1957:194).

It should be added that professions vary in the extent to which they are communities and exercise control over their members. The medical profession maintains stricter control over its members' practice than does an association of philosophers.

The image that seems to emerge from the professions is that their members are self-made people. Sacrifice, long hours of study, economic hardship, and delay of gratification have produced the present status of achievement. The skills one has developed are thus one's own personal property and are to be invested with the best possible return. Mercenary motives are eschewed. The professional presumes to know what is the common good and simultaneously projects an image of autonomy. Self-sacrifice and integrity are the basis for self or collegial self-regulation. Conditions of work, amount of fees, evaluation of deviations, diagnosis, and prescription are the professional's legitimate domain of autonomy. The image is that of competence bolstered by degrees, internships, previous employments, and licensure. Authority and respect are the side effects.

The professional community socializes its members into its own perspective in a variety of ways. When entering a profession, graduate training provides the contemporary role models, the reading lists of significant contributors, and the fellow students with whom one can develop one's competency. Licensure ensures that one is legitimated by society and fosters professional identity by defining acceptable roles and standards of excellence. A rich network of professional colleagues with similar interests, concerns, and priorities fosters the development of professional values and goals. Depending on the length of its history, the professional community can display its heroes to be imitated, as well as its fund of folk wisdom and objective information. Association with colleagues and immersion in the subject matter of the discipline results in a new language to describe reality, and a way of defining and resolving problems. The more coherent and integrated the professional community, the greater the expectations made of its members. If a professional group has a long history of status, or if it is presently fighting for a place in the occupations, it tends to be more exacting in its demands for conformity to the standards and ideology of the profession. Consequently, one cannot assume that the professional community is a neutral community. To uncritically accept the professional community as the context of one's work as a therapist is to make it one's primary frame of reference. Then there will be little conversation with the Christian community, much less any significant change.

However, professions as communities do not function in isolation. How does a particular profession relate to the larger culture? The professional community does not exist in a vacuum; society is the context. The relationship, however, is reciprocal. Society and profession are transformed by their mutual interaction. And if culture is ethical as argued earlier, then professions that reflect culture take on an ethical character as well. I begin with the society-to-profession movement of the dialectic.

First, the development of professions is limited to well-developed societies, regardless of political ideology. Both the nature and demands of such societies permit professions to flourish. The rationalized division of labor endemic to industrial societies requires problem-oriented experts who can experiment with means, systematize procedures, and formalize regulations. The professions provide the technicians. The tension, conflict, and anxiety common in highly competitive, work-oriented, status-seeking societies results in casualties; the professions then provide physical and emotional healers. With increasing variation in beliefs and lifestyle in pluralistic societies, traditional norms of right and wrong disappear; the professions provide the reality police to protect some of the sacred values. Society presents the needs and clientele; the professions in turn produce the therapists and managers.

Second, as the context of professional activities, societies shape not only what professionals do but also how they work. It should come as no great surprise that a society variously characterized as technological, market-oriented, and bureaucratic should influence the professions in the direction of technique, fees, and efficiency. It is in part from the surrounding culture that professions draw their modus operandi.

Third, society provides the fundamental values and the folk wisdom without which most professions could hardly exist. To be sure, each profession creates its own unique social reality, but unless there is congruence with the dominant values and beliefs of the larger culture, professions would be powerless. Moreover, given the gaps in our knowledge, professionals are forced to resort to commonsense wisdom contained in the heritage of a particular society. Society is then a critical source of basic values and beliefs on which professional activity is predicated.

Finally, society legitimates the professions. A paying, compliant clientele reinforces the rightful existence of the professional. Political sanction through state licensure blesses the activities of the "competent professional" in the eyes of the lay public. The evidence for such legitimation can be found in the prestige rankings society assigns to various professions.

The dialectic of professional and society applies to psychologists and therapists. Professional psychologists emerge out of society and at the same time uphold it. Goldstein (1973) has pointed out that for traditional psychotherapy the clients are primarily from middle-class social strata. Albee (1977) stated that psychology has a history of providing relief for emotional problems of the affluent. Often these are problems that emerge out of an industrial society. Or more specifically, the problems arise from the anxiety and guilt of a socially mobile class of people.

In turn, psychotherapy in its values and methods reflects the dominant culture. Over thirty years ago an analysis of mental health pamphlets (Gursslin, Hunt, and Roach, 1960) revealed that the focus was on such middle-class values as the virtue of work, controlling one's emotions, planning ahead, and achievement. Further, effective therapy requires clients who are self-reliant, are able to delay gratification, who are introspective and verbal. Even more explicitly, professional communities become ethical communities little different from religious bodies when they make pronouncements on issues from the Gulf War, abortion, and gay and lesbian rights. The professions are then communities of ethical discernment. Such pronouncements often disregard the diversity of opinion in the profession's membership. But it is inconsistent with the mandate the larger public gives to professional organizations. The task of professional community is to monitor adherence to a minimalist ethic and to ensure to the larger public that their members possess the skills they publicize.

Professions, Principalities, and Powers

Is there help in the New Testament for the Christian's understanding of such a social structure as the profession? Yes, I think there is, and it is located in the discussion of the "principalities and powers." Professions are social structures the New Testament community might have called a "power." My argument for this will rely heavily on the research of Hendrik Berkhof (1962) and Walter Wink (1984, 1986, 1992).

First, what is meant by the term "powers"? The term is borrowed from apocalyptic literature, where it referred to spiritual beings who influence human life. However, in the context of the expansion of the New Testament church into the Greco-Roman world it took on new meaning. Basing his argument on a variety of texts (Rom. 8:38; Col. 2:8; Gal. 4:1–3; Col. 1:15–17; Col. 2:13–15; Eph. 3:10), Berkhof concludes that the powers referred to all that orders human life, all that gave coherence, meaning, and structure. The powers continue to preserve the world from chaos. They are the structures we grew up with that gave our lives some measure of stability. The relevant texts assume that the powers include nature, spiritual beings, time, space, philosophy, the state, and the Jewish legal system.

The Christian's attitude toward these powers is ambivalent; they are both created and fallen. Their fallenness emerges when they assume too much, when they presume to provide meaning for all of life. In so doing they separate us from God, the ultimate source of life and meaning. In short, they become ends in themselves. The inevitable consequence is that they become oppressive. And it is in the death of Christ that their fallenness is revealed most clearly. Christ is crucified by the law of the Scribes, the temple cult of the priests, the piety of the Pharisees, the Roman law of Pilate. On the other hand, the powers are also seen as creative by the writer of the book to the Colossians. "He is the image of the invisible God, the firstborn over all creation. For by him all things are created: things in heaven and on earth, visible and invisible, whether thrones or powers or rules or authorities; all things are created by him and for him. He is before all things, and in him all things hold together" (Col. 1:15–17). Thus when the powers provide order, they do so by God's grace. When they are in subjection to Christ as Lord they can exercise their proper function—i.e., an instrumental role. But in order for this to occur they cannot be made sacred or absolute.

The relationship of the church to these powers is complex. When the powers are oppressive, the church may unmask them by the nature of its life or its direct witness. By confessing Christ as Lord, it sets limits to the comprehensiveness that a power may assume. The church is not called to destroy the powers. Rather, through the creation of a different social reality, it renders them less seductive. The power is only a part of creation, not all of reality. Nor is the church called to somehow make the powers Christian, for that strategy tends to underestimate the fallenness of the powers. It is through the church that "the manifold wisdom of God should be made known to the rulers and authorities in the heavenly places" (Eph. 3:10).

If we now apply the above sketch of the "principalities and powers" to the church and profession, the following implications arise. First, it is appropriate to view the church as a power. It provides a sense of order. It is susceptible to the temptation of taking itself too seriously, with the consequence that it too becomes oppressive. The experience of restriction that many a Christian has felt in the church may well be a result of ecclesiastical arrogance. After all, the church is only a sign of the Reign of God; it is not identical with the Reign of God. The church's goal as a fallen power is its own survival. But the church can also be a positive power. It is here that some of us first learned the stories of the Christian community, found role models for Christian maturity, and the importance of accountability. Many of us received a relatively coherent social world that continues to serve as a basis for personal growth. Most important is the fact that often the churches we came from had a sense of center, of identity. The church then was a power that provided order. Our churchly past deserves neither indiscriminate blessing nor wholesale condemnation.

The profession too is a power. It has given us gifts. Its pluralistic nature has in fact encouraged tolerance of many points of view, including religious ones. Furthermore, the mental health profession has forced the church to deal with issues it has neglected, such as physical and sexual abuse. It has provided careful analysis of the human self in the modern world. On the other hand, the profession as a community, by virtue of its gift of pluralism, lacks a center, a point of transcendence. It becomes a mosaic of "villages" and reifies the search for truth as truth itself. The secular profession assumes that the individual possesses the resources to make meaningful and just decisions. The locus of moral authority is then grounded only in reason, nature, or history.

One last point. Berkhof makes a comment that is relevant here. He observes that, with respect to the powers (read professions), Christians tend to oscillate between two extremes. At one extreme there is an uncritical acceptance of the powers in structuring our life. At the other extreme there is despair over our ability to get out from under the oppression of the powers in our society. Both are errors. The first is too romantic. It underestimates the ability of the powers or professions to separate us from God. The second position fails to recognize the lordship of Christ in the presence of unjust powers or professions. It is too pessimistic.

Vocation without Ethical Discernment

Professionalization is a process encountered by most individuals who seek to become mental health practitioners. There is an additional question that the Christian as therapist faces. What is the relation of one's professional activities to one's faith? The notion that is often used to interpret and legitimate one's work is that of "calling." The logic is as follows. God calls Christians to various positions in society to be a light to the world. To the extent that Christians fill vacant offices, the Christian has an opportunity to exert influence in the direction of his or her values. It is assumed that each little light will eventually result in a transformation of society. The courage to continue is rooted in the call that God has given the individual for a particular station in the occupational structure of society. Thus it is not uncommon to hear Christians say that God has called them to work in the area of psychology, for example.

Historically, a shift took place in the understanding of the nature of the Christian's calling. While in the New Testament that call is interpreted within the context of the Christian community, progressively the calling was applied more to occupations generally. A noticeable change occurred in the Constantinian era. With the identification of the church with the state, antagonism toward the Christian was removed, as was a transcendent view of society. John Howard Yoder points out,

> Since there are no more confessing heathen, every profession must be declared Christian. Since Christian norms for the exercise of some professions are difficult to find, the norms of pagan *justicia* will be declared to define the content of Christian love. The autonomy of the state and the other realms of culture are not brought concretely under the lordship of Christ, with a total revision of form and content which that would involve; it has been baptized while retaining its former content (1960:22).

In the Middle Ages, the world, as it was for first-century Christians, was dark and foreboding. Anything associated with the world, including work, was irrevocably evil. Not surprisingly, the monastic movement emerged. Calling was then limited specifically to churchly vocations. The change in the meaning of calling during the Reformation was in response to this limited definition. Luther reacted strongly: "the orders of pope,

bishop, priest and monk are sinful orders" (Wingren, 1957:3).
For Luther the world was not in a state of chaos because of the
fall. Instead the world was orderly and predictable. The
church-world dichotomy was again abandoned and in its place
we have Christian institutions such as marriage and government. All of these institutions belong to God's created order,
including the military. It is from God that the soldier receives
his fitness to do battle. The cobbler too is doing God's work.
The secular domain was again made sacred. Ellul (1974) sum-
marizes it well when he states:

> He who performed a particular profession did so because he was
> called upon by God to hold *that* particular profession, and not
> another. Each individual entered into God's design in a partic-
> ular way. There is no longer a *general* calling for work, but a
> unique calling addressed to each individual to become a brick-
> layer, or a doctor, etc. This brings about, on the one hand, the
> impossibility of thoroughly classifying the professions which
> please God, and those which are cursed. . . . On the other hand,
> the individual assumes the responsibility that each person must
> ask himself: What type of work does God wish me to do? (25).

Given the earlier analysis of the profession's intimate relation to society, I can hardly endorse the notion of calling when
it is applied to a profession. The professional role is only one
among many roles a Christian may assume. The Christian is
called to be a member of the Reign of God and not primarily of
any one professional community. The call involves an individual response to Jesus as Lord and Savior. That individual is
committed to the extension of that community as a sign of
God's activity in history. The Reign of God is the overarching
context of our work in the world. It is this call that gives the
individual Christian a sense of identity and purpose. The Reign
of God, when it manifests itself in the life of the church, is the
locus of our responsibility and accountability.

On the other hand, just as the profession has been an escape
for some disenchanted religious professionals, so also exclusive
involvement in the life of the church has been used by some
professionals as an evasion of serious involvement in the issues
and needs of society. Perhaps one of the reasons professionalism has become such a problem is because the church itself has
bought into professionalism. Pastors who preach in the spe-

cialized jargon of theology are little different than professional psychologists who parade their vocabulary. The way we organize our church life at times differs little from organizational charts of large bureaucracies. We have become as growth conscious as most financial organizations. When we assume that God is no larger than the perspective of our community, then we are as provincial as some warring ethnoreligious groups.

In order to justify their work as Christian, some therapists have utilized the notion of individual calling. The occupational structure of Western society is then reified. It becomes a given. One tends to overlook the relationship of the profession to the larger social context when calling is interpreted in a very individual sense. By virtue of the individualism of some professionals, there is really no visible structure of accountability. The social vacuum is filled by the profession to which God has called one. The norms are not self-consciously derived from the Reign of God. The roles that these occupations impose on the individual and the appropriate activities are accepted as part of the calling. Calling, then, becomes a legitimation of the cultural milieu. The assessment of culture is then less clear. The ideology of the professions becomes that of the Christian professional.

I would propose an identity not based on career. In order to develop such an identity, there must be a significant group other than the professional community as a point of reference. I submit that that group is the fellowship of brothers and sisters who seek to incarnate the ethic of the Reign of God. What are the implications for the professional who wishes to make the churchly community the center of personal identity? What are the consequences for a church that seeks to provide a home for professionals?

The church can affirm gifts and abilities. If the church is a significant community, its involvement is not limited to that time when the training is completed and one has already entered into a specific occupation. The church is the context in which abilities can be tested. In the New Testament church such testing involved the discernment of gifts and the approval for a specific ministry by the laying on of hands.

Unfortunately, selection of a profession is increasingly left to the preferences, interests, or even whims of the individual. We urge young people to choose what fits, or we give vocational interest inventories so one can compare patterns of interests with professionals already on the job. But the fact that my unique history of experiences has produced a set of abilities that match that of an engineer, lawyer, or teacher, is hardly sufficient reason to enter any one of those professions. Moreover, this process takes the types of occupations available in our society as given. In contrast, the church must take seriously the likelihood that some work may be inappropriate for Christians and some work more consistent with the needs of society as perceived by the church. Is the need for mental health professionals in the West as pressing as it is in underdeveloped countries?

The task of the church then is to develop a sense of priorities in service and to assist in the discernment of abilities. Abdication of this responsibility of the church reinforces the notion that selection of an occupation depends only on the choice of the individual.

The focus of this chapter has been on the role of the professional community vis-à-vis the church community. I have argued that church community is the locus of accountability, and that professions tend to assume independence and autonomy. They develop a morality of their own. Members are expected to be accountable to the professional society over other groups. The professional community has knowledge and a perspective on certain issues that presumably the lay person cannot understand. Hence, for the church to presume it has something to say is often perceived as meddling.

Christian professionals who make the church their primary community of ethical discernment are accountable to their brothers and sisters. My functioning in a particular profession affects the witness of the church to the human community. Not only is the church the locus of accountability, it is quite capable of responding on ethical matters once the issues are explained. The ethical issues of abortion and euthanasia can be examined with other Christians. Patient and client rights can be discussed with profit by people who are often on the receiving end of the professional services. The church can then be a center of accountability and discernment in ethical issues. It is not merely one more group in which the professional is a member. These are the professional's "people." To take that seriously means that one seeks to involve the church in the problems faced by professionals. The problem of one person in the church is a problem for all.

On the other side, trained professionals can assist the church in its ministries and bring to bear professional expertise that enables the church to be more faithful. I have seen professionals who have been sensitive to the vision of the church and who have offered their skills in administration, counseling, or education. In the relationship of the church to the profession there is then a place for each to critique the other, to listen quietly, to accept correction, to wrestle with problems, and to forgive errors. Conflict between church and profession is inevitable when the profession assumes absolute commitment or when the church presumes that its life completely reflects the Reign of God.

The Church as Secondary Ethical Community

When the profession is the exclusive ethical community for the professional therapist who is also a Christian, then the church is simply a community that may provide a set of friends or some additional clients. The church will not become a community of ethical discourse if it is viewed from strictly a utilitarian perspective by therapists. The utilitarian view is as follows. The church is useful to the therapist. It can prayerfully support one's work. It can provide a substantial pool of clients and it can legitimate one's "calling" as a "Christian psychologist." The church can provide facilities in which therapy can occur. This reduces expense and increases profits. It may give one a forum in which to express ideas through Sunday school and weekend seminars. Some of these practices may be good, but from the point of view of the utilitarian ethic, they first satisfy the professional needs of the therapist to establish a practice in a familiar and productive setting. Is it possible that the church, as an ethically discerning community, has more to give? When the church engages in the process of ethical reflection as a body, it serves an even more important function. *By its story and life it gives content to the moral language that is the foundation of the therapeutic event.*

The church serves another function for the therapist when it becomes solely a community of personal emotional support. Through its liturgy, its sacraments, and its life, the therapist is personally revitalized for ministry. This is the place where one can express how one feels. It is the place where one is understood. It is a community of like-minded Christians who come from a similar socioeconomic status. Bellah and his associates (1985) point out that when communities are developed in an individualistic society, they are "life-style enclaves." They are groups of people with very similar interests and from similar professions. The church can become a lifestyle enclave for the therapist. Too often the church becomes only a community of emotional support. To be sure, such support happens less often than it should. Nonetheless, the church is also called to be a community of righteousness in the midst of society. Emotional support is in conjunction with that enterprise, not a substitute. A community that has no consensus about its moral vocabulary and no consensus on its praxis also will not provide the therapist with human examples of the values he or she espouses in therapy.

The Professional and the Christian Community

The Christian community as ethical community may collaborate with professional therapists. How then do we do so? The first question the church must address to itself is: To what extent does the church reflect the social context in which it is situated? When this question is answered, the church can assist the professional with the same issue. To the extent that the church seeks genuinely to reflect the New Testament model of the Reign of God, to that extent it will be less likely to be captive to any power.

A church community that is able to address the powers recognizes that the Reign of God is the primary story. As the church becomes a sign of the Reign of God it can become increasingly a primary community of personal identity, accountability, and ethical discernment. It is here in the Christian community that the implications of Christ's lordship for our work in the professions are tested out. In the community of ethical discernment the extent to which a profession has become a creative or fallen power is determined. Then profession can be a usable social structure that is not given ultimate power.

Allow me to suggest a direction such a discernment might take. Banks (1983) makes an interesting comparison between caring in first-century Hellenistic and Jewish communities. In both, mutual aid was assumed to be at the heart of community life. Voluntary associations abounded to satisfy needs from burial to social support. However, in the Greek communities the principle of mutual financial, personal, and social support was a carefully regulated affair and kept within strictly calculated limits. In this respect it mirrored the practice of philanthropy at this time in general. It worked on the principle of reciprocal return: those who gave expected something in response, loyalty perhaps, or assistance in their various causes.

In Jewish/Christian circles, donors gave physical and social aid because they had received freely from God's own hands. This was rooted historically in the Exodus event of liberation and contemporaneously in the gift of God through synagogue life. The motive was personal and communal gratitude for the experience of the salvation of God in Christ (2 Cor. 8:9ff). Furthermore, the aid was unobtrusively given without discrimination (1 Cor. 1:26; Matt. 4:46; Mark 2:17; Rom. 5:6; 2 Cor. 5:14–16). Third, the care was given to the point of sacrifice (2 Cor. 2:3–4; 1 Thess. 2:8; 2 Cor. 5:14–16; 1 Cor. 12:23). And lastly, every aspect of life was ministered to: physical, material, personal, and social (2 Cor. 12:10; 14:1–5, 30). Banks concludes that the Jewish communities modeled a new dimension of care.

Professions are powers. They may provide real services to individuals in need, or they may seek to perpetuate themselves at all costs. When professions disseminate knowledge and information rather than creating a monopoly on it, they are a positive power. When there are clear lines of accountability, when clients are not made dependent, when professionals admit their limitations in knowledge and skill, when they provide services regardless of race, class, or creed, then a profession can be trusted as a power. But when professions create marketable needs, mechanically exercise skills without compassion, exact exorbitant fees, or avoid public scrutiny, they become a fallen power that is self-serving and coercive.

The ideal response of the church to professions need not be either black or white, acceptance or rejection. Sometimes the stance of the individual Christian or of the church may be that of a listener in a dialogue where neither has the answer (e.g., the best system of welfare) and in which both partners have something to learn. Or, one can take on the role of translator. Then one attempts to translate language of the profession for the members of the church or vice versa. In his day the apostle Paul translated the Hebrew-Christian vision into the language understandable by the Greeks. In other settings, we may appear no different than other professionals who do not make the same, or any, profession of faith. Whether a Christian or secular psychologist runs a statistical analysis, the conclusions are not more sound if conducted by the former. Another chapter will examine these positions in greater detail.

There may be times when we as Christians engaged in professional endeavors may need to clearly distance ourselves from the theory, practice, or position of a profession. This is specifically the case when the profession becomes an oppressive power. For example, the fragmentation of communities in North American culture may encourage an individualism that some psychologists then bless as self-actualization. The degeneration of personal relationships may be reflected in a fee-for-service relationship of therapist and client. The technological mentality of some professionals is often translated into models of pragmatic, behavior-modifying therapies. The conflict between the various "villages" in North American culture is reflected in the implicit racism in some psychological theories of intelligence.

Professions and disciplines such as psychology become absolute in several ways. Psychologists begin by failing or even refusing to recognize the relationship of their theory-building to the historical context in which it occurs. To the extent that psychologists perceive themselves as ahistorical, they can then argue that their findings are value-free or transhistorical. Implicit in this ahistorical position, however, is a strong political stance that supports the status quo. As a result, the basic postulates and conclusions of psychological methodology and research reflect the prevailing culture. Unable to provide a critique, psychologists can become unconscious supporters of an oppressive system and fail to liberate the depressed or the oppressed.

Professionalism, when it makes the profession the primary community of ethical discernment, makes it difficult to take the Christian community seriously as a primary ethical community. It will demand of us a new kind of professionalism, but not a rejection of professional competence. It will require a recovery of a vision of the church as discerning community. If we expect the church and the Christian therapist to be sensitive to the oppression experienced by the disabled, women, and the poor then the church must reflect on its praxis. Where the church has failed it can repent and develop a practice consistent with its own story. Where the church has been faithful, it has reason to be grateful.

7

A Community of Discernment

In the previous chapter I examined the relationship of the mental health professional to the Christian community. In this chapter I wish to illustrate the way the Christian community can converse with the professional community. The former becomes a significant ethical community when it discerns the meaning of the Reign of God in the society in which it exists and assists its members in reflecting on ways in which their work is an extension of the Reign of God.

The church's response to professionalism can be one of discernment or wooden positioning. Throughout the history of Christianity, the church has responded in many ways to societal structures. Sometimes that response was one of rejection of culture as pagan, while at other times it was one of uncritical acceptance of professionalism as a gift. There is a range of intermediate strategies. Any strategy that leads to consistent and complete rejection of the profession or identification with it is problematic. The work of Robert Banks (1980, 1987) has been most helpful in understanding the church's role interpreting the nature of work and its relationship to the faith community.

Not only does the church vacillate between absolute rejection or acceptance, it also tends to freeze one specific response proper at one point in history as the approach appropriate for all cultures in all times. While it may be appropriate to be very reject-

149

ing of an aspect of culture at one time in history, it might be appropriate to be more accepting at another because conditions have changed. The thesis of this chapter is that there are a variety of appropriate strategies for the dialogue between church and profession, and that exclusive use of a single strategy is of limited value. Whatever the strategy to be used, we will need to be sensitive to the specific psychological issue being addressed. Different responses are appropriate depending on whether we are relating scientific research, archetypal images, or systems theory to the Christian story. I submit that the nature of the specific psychological issue needs, in part, to inform our specific religious response. My intention is to illustrate a variety of approaches as legitimate. This chapter will pursue the dialogue by explaining five historic approaches to culture in general and applying them to the profession of psychology in particular. The five approaches will be seen as metaphors (Barbour, 1974). This chapter is my attempt at nuancing the term "integration." The dialogue can take many forms.

Strategies of Interaction: An Overview

In his classic treatment of the relationship of Christ and culture, Niebuhr (1951) delineates five strategies of interaction. The first type (sectarian) assumes a fundamental discontinuity between Christ and culture. All of culture is viewed as pagan, and hence any interaction presumably will result in compromise. Niebuhr rejected this strategy because cultural isolation and irrelevance of the church were then inevitable. The second strategy (nineteenth-century liberalism) assumes an essential continuity between the ethic of Jesus and the highest ideals of human civilization. Niebuhr pointed out that a critique of culture by the church is thereby rendered impossible. A third strategy (Thomistic) assumes a valid contribution of culture but asserts that Christ is above culture. This position, in Niebuhr's estimation, too easily baptizes as Christian one aspect of culture and thus opens itself to the charge of provincialism. Another strategy (Lutheran) assumes that Christ and culture are irreconcilable and that they must be held in tension. Such a strategy, says Niebuhr, fails to provide a basis on which the church has a unique contribution to make to society and hence tends too easily to support the status quo.

A last position (Reformed) proposes that the relationship between Christ and culture is one of transformation. Culture can be converted and used to the glory of God. This appears to be Niebuhr's nomination for the most appropriate strategy since he submitted no critique of it.

In contrast to Niebuhr, my focus is not on culture as a monolithic entity but as a composite of specific actions, beliefs, traditions, and communities. It is not then something that one either totally accepts, rejects, or transforms. Next, I will focus on the implications for professionalism, one community in the larger culture. Third, I will focus on the church's (rather than Niebuhr's primary focus on Christ's) response to culture/professionalism (Yoder, 1964). It is the church as the symbolic presence of Jesus in the world that encounters the various dimensions of culture, including the mental health profession.

What follows is an adaptation of Niebuhr's typology. These strategies for interaction between faith and profession will be reconstructed so that, on the one hand, we protect the integrity of the vision of the Reign of God, and, on the other hand, we trust that there are dimensions of culture that are good and useful in the work of the church. Each of the following strategies is also a role an individual Christian can play within the mental health professions. Each will be developed in greater detail below.

1. *Critique.* No profession can go unquestioned by a Christian who takes seriously the transcendence of God and the normativity of the Reign of God. Uncritical incorporation of disciplinary insights is not an acceptable option. The more difficult task is that of developing criteria and categories by which one judges a specific contribution.

2. *Consistency.* The encounter of the church and the profession is not automatically one of withdrawal. There are continuities or consistencies. Where we find genuine freedom, reconciliation, and care consistent with the Reign of God, there we gratefully acknowledge God's presence in action. Though the consistency is always partial, it is nevertheless a similarity of cultures and points to affirmation.

3. *Translation.* The vision of the church and the mandate of a profession are couched in language. There have

been numerous attempts at translation. Thus it is appropriate to ask how the Christian message can be translated into the language of mental health professionals and vice versa.

4. *Dialogue.* If we recognize that God is at work in the world of both believer and unbeliever, then it is entirely appropriate for us to take the posture of listener in the dialogue of faith and profession. Whether we, in Western culture, are Christians or not, we face some of the same problems (Palmer, 1988). Cannot the observations of those who are not Christians help Christians in their efforts to be faithful?

5. *Witness.* There is a point where the therapist with Christian convictions has a distinct contribution to make to the conversation. This contribution is not a response that emerges from an attitude of imperialism as it is a point to truth beyond ourselves. It assumes that there is Good News and that the human dilemma is in some way related to a rejection of it.

Critique

The Strategy

This position assumes that Christ is against culture. It "uncompromisingly affirms the sole authority of Christ over the Christian and resolutely rejects culture's claims to loyalty" (Niebuhr 1951:45). Niebuhr grants that such a view follows logically from the Christian principle of the lordship of Jesus Christ and that it is an attitude typical of Christians in the early church. In the first letter of John one finds both an emphasis on obedience to the commandment of Jesus Christ (2:3–11) and also a rejection of the "world": "Do not love the world or the things in the world. If anyone loves the world, love for the Father is not in him" (1 John 2:15). Niebuhr assumes that "world" for the writer meant the whole society outside the church, which in turn implied that Christians were called to reject culture. The world is under the realm of the power of evil, dominated by the "lust of the flesh, the lust of the eyes and the pride of life" (1 John 2:16). The world is transitory, and our loyalty should be directed toward the new order of the Lord Jesus Christ. Niebuhr assumes that since the writer expected the immanent return of Christ and the end of the world, there was no need for instructions about participation in social institutions.

In the church of the first centuries after Christ, similar attitudes can be found. Tertullian presents Christianity as a way of life quite separate from culture, with more emphasis on law and obedience than on grace. There are two ways, one of life and one of death. There is a radical separation of the Christian and the non-Christian. Jesus remains the absolute authority and requires obedience to his commandments: love of brother and enemy, nonresistance to evil, prohibitions of anger and the lustful look. On the other hand, the Christian is to shun the pagan world with its idolatrous religion and withdraw from occupations contrary to the spirit of Christ (e.g., public meetings, military service, business). For Tertullian there are no positive connections between the faith of Christians and the philosophy of the Greeks. Whatever truth there is to be found there can also be derived from the Scriptures.

Throughout the history of the church there have been individuals and groups, according to Niebuhr, who "have felt themselves compelled by loyalty to Christ to withdraw from culture and to give up all responsibility for the world" (57). For him these include the medieval monastic movement, the Anabaptist Mennonites, Tolstoy, Kierkegaard, and sectarian Protestantism. All have in common the acknowledgment of the sole authority of Jesus Christ and the common rejection of the prevailing culture, which is always seen as pagan and corrupt. The old order is passing away and is to be judged by the emerging new order. In evaluating this position, Niebuhr finds it a necessary but inadequate answer to the question of the relation of Christ and culture. It is necessary because in the past it has maintained a distinction between Christ and Caesar, between revelation and reason, and between God's will and ours. True, monasticism became a transmitter of cultural tradition—not only religious vision—and Protestant sectarians made a contribution to such political customs as religious liberty for all members of society. But these contributions were indirect. It has required others of different persuasions on the Christ-culture question to work out the implications.

Application

My adaptation of this strategy is to argue that critique is one (but only one) of the church's responses to culture and professionalism. It is appropriate for any scholar or professional to be critical of one's chosen discipline. However, what is needed is a more discerning response than the fundamentalist's rejection of professional psychology. The issue is which aspects of the profession should be rejected. This is not a rejection *en toto*. Rather, this stance refuses to accept the sense of autonomy that human institutions as fallen "powers" tend to claim for themselves. Theoretical systems that make a claim to universality, professional groups that claim our primary allegiance, or therapeutic approaches that presume exclusiveness of technique need the humility that comes with a commitment to the Reign of God. When made absolute, theories, practices, and communities become destructive.

The strategy of critique assumes a point of departure that transcends culture and tradition from which to interpret professional communities. For the Christian it is the truth of the Reign of God to which the church witnesses. While we recognize that God's revelation occurs in history, it is a fundamental assumption that God transcends history and tradition and chooses to be revealed in human culture. Where aspects of culture presume that transcendence, there is a clear conflict. Where this is the case, challenge, rejection, and withdrawal are legitimate responses.

A critique of the mental health and psychological professions is consistent with this historic response of the church to culture. What would be the nature of such a critique? The following might be some directions worth pursuing. For example, we should have spoken a resounding "No!" rather than assist in the A-bomb testing during the 1950s, and wherever today our work assists in the destruction of human life. A psychological theory of education or development that proposes, assumes, or supports racism deserves critique. The individualism implicit in a wide array of contemporary psychological theories simply ignores our responsibility to live in accountability (Wallach and Wallach, 1983). A developmental psychology that implicitly takes the prevailing culture as the final goal of development desperately needs a critical appraisal of social realities (Peck,

1987). A behaviorism that cannot appreciate the elements of mystery in personality fails to recognize the image of God in humankind. A therapy that considers acceptance and nondirectiveness as primary may be antinomian and inimical to the development of tradition (May, Rogers, and Maslow, 1986). In each case the fundamental critique is against a sacrifice of transcendence for immanence.

The limitation of this strategy of critique, when it is not complemented by other strategies developed below, is that the more systemic the critique, the more easily the Christian professional lapses into cynicism and withdrawal. Critique is no justification for isolation from professionalism, only for action more consistent with one's convictions as they emerge from a consciousness shaped by the Reign of God.

Consistency

The Strategy

This strategy of relating church and culture/profession assumes there is more continuity than discontinuity. Whereas the first strategy says "no," this strategy says "yes." This position includes persons who count themselves believers who are yet inclusive and ecumenical in their relationship with all other believers. They feel equally at home in the church and in the world of culture. Niebuhr (1951) indicates that for these people there is no felt tension "between church and world, social laws and Gospel, divine grace and human effort, the ethics of salvation and the ethics of social conservation or progress" (83).

One very clear biblical example of this position is found in the wisdom literature of the Old Testament. This literature assumes that proverbs have universal application and that their source is to be found in the larger human community. There is none of the particularism of the first strategy here. Wisdom is collected from a variety of Near Eastern cultures and incorporated into the life of God's people. If the wisdom is consistent with the story of Yahweh's people, it is acceptable.

In this strategy Niebuhr indicates that "Christ is identified with what men conceive to be their finest ideals, their noblest institutions, and their best philosophy" (103). Also, this position, in Niebuhr's estimation, has contributed to the extension of Christ's power over humanity. By finding likeness between Jesus and Socrates or the deaths of Christ and of Gandhi, we make clear the presence of God in history. This position seeks to make apparent the universal meaning of the Gospel. Jesus is not simply the savior of a small band of followers but of the whole world.

Application

In contrast to the strategy of critique, the argument for consistency points to continuity rather than discontinuity. It assumes a correlation in the attributes of the objects compared. Any comparison will contain some points of similarity and some points of dissimilarity. After two millennia of existence, there is a residual effect of Christianity even in what has been referred to as a post-Christian era. The worlds of art, politics, welfare, and mental health have all been affected in varying degrees by the Judeo-Christian heritage. Those continuities can be affirmed when they are filtered through the vision of the Christian community. In the past this strategy tended to be an apologetic that made Christianity attractive and relevant. In my proposal, this strategy is an attempt to acknowledge those values, beliefs, and practices in the profession that are consistent with the story of the Reign of God.

A fundamental assumption of this strategy is that God works in the life of both the church and the profession, the believer and the unbeliever, among Jews and Gentiles. It is then entirely possible that one might find some similarities—though rough in some cases—between the words and acts of God and the words and acts of humanity. This approach begins with the fact of God's self-disclosure and then moves by comparison from God's covenant to creation, from God's action to ours, from the Christ event to historical events. Human love then takes on meaning in the light of God's sacrificial love in Jesus Christ, our peacemaking in the light of God's acts of reconciliation. Where it is apparent that there is a clear, though partial, correspondence between the message of Christianity and that of various voices of culture, our response can be one of grateful acknowledgment and acceptance.

Using the concept of "analogy of faith," Thomas Oden (1966) has selected the area of therapy and explored its implications. He points to the following consistencies: The counselor who is immersed in the frame of reference of the troubled person, thereby obtaining an understanding of the person, reflects the fact that God in Jesus Christ understands who we are. In both cases there is an entry into the estrangement of the other. Such involvement is not passive but radically active. The therapist who participates in the estrangement of the client without losing a sense of identity echoes God's participation in our estrangement. The therapist who is faced with hostility, guilt, and anxiety, and still identifies with the client, parallels God's identification with us. In both there is an element of engagement and separation. The therapist who accepts the client reflects God's acceptance of us and our inadequacies. The therapist who does not condemn mirrors God's forgiveness of our transgressions. The counselor who creates a permissive environment in which a client can begin to exercise self-direction models God's grace to us as we seek to grow in faithfulness. In both, healing is seen as a gift that emerges from beyond ourselves. If, in the process of therapy, an individual begins to move outward to others with genuine interest because of the unconditional love of the therapist, then that therapist's actions are analogous to those acts of love and care God shows toward us.

The strategy of finding continuity is, like the others developed in this chapter, limited and best used in conjunction with the others. Analogy is not total parity or disparity. To compare two objects, ideas, or events is to assume that they are neither totally similar nor totally different. To use the notion of *consistency* in talking about God and culture is to assume that they are neither univocal nor equivocal. However, the problem endemic to this strategy is the tendency toward equation. If one begins with a weak view of God's self-disclosure to us, the use of consistency degenerates into deriving hard conclusions about God's nature from natural processes and relationships. The therapist is clearly bound by cultural condition, personal weaknesses, and conflicts.

The Christian community is the context in which correspondences are evaluated. Metaphors and actions vary in their consistency with the Reign of God, and hence discernment is necessary. Unless the church expends the energy to reflect on the analogies between God's actions in history and our efforts to be therapeutic, the time will come when we will simply assume there is no difference, or even, to ask the question will be irrelevant.

Translation

The Strategy

If the first position completely separates Christ and culture and the second accommodates one to the other, the third position seeks to synthesize Christ and culture while maintaining a hierarchical distinction between the two. In part, the juxtaposition of Christ's humanity and divinity would be an example of the mindset of this strategy.

The best representative of this position is, of course, Thomas Aquinas. Aquinas spoke as one who was a member of a church that had become guardian of culture. Here the church has accepted full social responsibility for society, the family, and religion. It is this social unification of Church and society that was made explicit in Aquinas's theological and philosophical synthesis. His system was an architectonic structure that incorporated philosophy and theology, state and church, natural and divine laws, Christ and culture. He accepted the Aristotelianism of his day and assumed that the Creator of nature and the immanent spirit are identical. On the basis of reason it is apparent, says Aquinas, that all nature is purposive in character, and on the basis of faith we know that this purpose is fulfilled in God alone. Aquinas accepted the Aristotelian analysis of reality and found the complement in Christianity. The former was the way of culture, of moral training in good habits and intelligent self-direction. The latter, however, comes only with divine assistance, a happiness that finds its source in the supernatural. The foundation is the natural, and the supernatural is then added. The order of the natural is discernible through reason, while the supernatural is given by faith. The natural order may change from era to era, but the laws of God are unchanging and implicit in nature, for nature is created by God. The institutions of society are to be governed by natural reason, while the church directs the individual to supernatural ends. This hierarchy then provides an organic interdependence of higher and lower but still guards the independence of each. In this approach, what is right is discovered in the given, created nature of the person and of the world; ought is derived from what is created.

Application

The application of this approach to relating psychology and Christianity might be referred to as a process of translation. In part, Aquinas translated Aristotelian concepts into Christianity. The role of the translator assumes two rather coherent language systems, each with its own unique vocabulary, rules of grammar, and perspectives on reality. Faced with a mosaic of languages, confusion in communication, and the absence of good translations, a linguist sets about the task of immersion in language study, cultural analysis, and translation. The linguist is in the position of choosing an expression that will best communicate an idea in the original language. Hence, translations vary in their ability to communicate.

Translation as an activity is not confined to linguistic fields, but applies to other communities as well. The church as a discerning community is engaged in a process of translating its story for the professional community. In some ways translating Hebrew into Greek is like translating the vision of Jerusalem into the cultural meanings of Athens, of the Reign of God into that of modernity. Moreover, the metaphor "translation" assumes that one is translating from the known to the unknown. It is assumed that the issue is not metaphysical or religious reality, but choosing and testing the best language to communicate a vision. The process of translation is intuitive, cognitive, and empirical. The adequacy of a translation is tested in terms of both its intuitive sense of fit and its rational consistency. Empirically a translation can be tested by its consequences for the life of the community.

A variety of languages have been developed to describe the person. We can do so at the biochemical level, seeing stress as secretion of digestive hormones into the stomach with subsequent ulceration. Or we can use the language of neurology and interpret thinking in terms of brain processes. Or we can use the language of theology and interpret learning with the vocabulary of conditioning, imprinting, reflexes, patterns of reinforcement, and the learning environment. We can use the terminology of scientific psychology and employ the naturalistic concepts of cause and effect, regression analysis, controlled observation and manipulation of variables, and operational definitions. Cognition can be examined using the lexicology of computer technology: input, storage, buffers, retrieval, networks, and organization. All of these languages have in common the fact that, fundamentally, natural metaphors are being used.

Historical metaphors are as common in psychological accounts as naturalistic ones. Some advocate that autobiography is the quintessential mode of understanding human nature. Others use historical change as the organizing motif: developmental or stage theories and age-related changes in behavior and dialectical development. Some use the language of decision: action, consequences, reflexiveness, responsibility, and change. One can also use the language of the sociologist: roles, institutionalization, alienation, authority, tradition, class, rationalization, or status. And one can use the glossary of cultural anthropologists to examine human behavior in terms of mores, symbols, evolution, kinship, national character, adaptation, taboos, sanctions, ritual, and acculturation.

Somewhere between the natural and the historical systems are the uniquely psychological metaphors. Structuralism focuses on consciousness, introspection, experience, attention, sensations, apperception, and chronometry. Functionalist language uses another vocabulary: adaptation, adjustment, evolution, individual differences, drives, and problem solving. Then, of course, there is the dictionary of terms provided by behaviorism: stimulus, response reinforcement, conditioning, behavior, association, conditional response, environmentalism, shaping, and spontaneous recovery. Phenomenology develops yet another set of terms: gestalt, context, qualities, holism, and closure. Even field theory in physics has been employed to explain individual behavior: forces, topology, equilibrium, tension-systems, valence, life-space, locomotion, and permeable boundaries.

The possible responses of the Christian professional as linguist to this plethora of languages are several. First, there is the simple recognition of the diversity of languages available for describing human behavior. Second, one can guard against making absolute any one language as the only or best language for mental health practice. Reductionism is a besetting sin of theoretical pursuits. Third, one can compare languages to determine the relative strengths and weaknesses of a particular symbol system: what aspect of human reality is slighted?

how consistent is the theory in its proposals? what is the fundamental metaphor that gives coherence to a particular symbol system? how is it different from other languages? in what contexts are some languages more appropriate than others? While all languages listed above describe human reality, some focus on one aspect of that reality with greater intensity and provide greater differentiation. For example, one theory may be especially sensitive to the dimension of freedom, action, responsibility, and self-consciousness. Other theories may be more suitable to an analysis of committed relationships, friendship, tradition, and culture.

But in addition to appropriateness of context and focus, are there any other ways of testing the usefulness of a particular language? If the Christian community is the context for the process of translation, one can ask about the consistency of any language with that of the Christian community, and one can ask whether a particular language leads to community and whether a particular language leads to greater faithfulness to the ethic of the Reign of God.

Ultimately, the test of the adequacy of a language is its effect on the way of living of an individual or of the human community. A language system that inspires greater acts of justice, kindness, liberation, joy, and forgiveness is a useful language or theory. However, the criteria are derived from a point other than the language itself. The usual test of language is its correspondence to physical reality. When there is an acceptable level of correspondence we say the theory is true. But there are other ways of viewing truth than the Greek way. The Hebrews tended to test the truth of a statement by its ability to inspire truthful actions.

A number of attempts have been made, by those who have theological concerns and psychological interests, to translate the language of Christianity into a particular social science theory. Some have translated Christianity into the language of scientific psychology (Myers, 1978), existential psychology (Tweedie, 1961), transactional psychology (Malony, 1979), psychoanalysis (Tillich, 1964), Jungian psychology (Cox, 1959), and Rogerian nondirective therapy (Browning, 1966).

Thus one of the strategies of the psychologist who is Christian can include taking a particular psychological theory and translating the terms as best one can. Oden (1966), for example, has translated theological language into that of nondirective therapy. Sin is translated as incongruence, introjected values, and conditions of worth. Redemption is viewed as congruence, empathy, and unconditional positive regard. Growth in grace becomes openness to experience, congruence—the fully functioning person.

David Myers (1978) attempts to translate aspects of the Christian message into the language of scientific psychology. He justified this by stating that

> the historic Hebrew-Christian view sees God acting and revealing himself through all events of his creation. The Spirit of God is understood as something greater than merely another force which sometimes intervenes in nature. Christians can therefore see psychological research in Christian terms as exploration of the natural revelation (256).

The Hebrew assumption that the person is a unity is translated into the scientific language of psychosomatic unity. The Jewish-Christian view of the relationship of thought and action is translated into research findings that demonstrate that "we are as likely to act ourselves into a way of thinking as to think ourselves into acting" (Myers, 1978:268). The tension between divine sovereignty and human responsibility is translated into the language of environmental control and personal responsibility.

One attempt to examine the relationship between the language of the Believers' Church tradition and that of a particular model of mental health services was developed by Myron Ebersole (1961). Ebersole focused on the conceptual model of the "therapeutic community." It provided "a theoretical basis for their [the mental health professional's] interest in creating a primary group context of concern and trust in which clients could feel some confidence to reassume responsibility for their own attitudes and behavior" (48). In contrast to prevailing practices, the approach assumed less hierarchical structure, less formalized patterns of communication, broader participation in decision making, and conscious use of the setting for treatment. Such an approach is consistent with a Believers' Church perspective on the nature of the Christian community and the importance of voluntary individual responsibility. The individual is seen in relational terms rather than individualistically. Yet Ebersole did not assume parity between church and the notion of therapeutic community. The church is a community of devotion and has more permanent and holistic purposes. The therapeutic community has the more limited goal of finding resources to begin moving toward mental health. though it is entirely possible that a patient might move on to participate in a community of devotion. To attempt to get a patient in therapy to incorporate new doctrinal beliefs may be both counterproductive and unethical.

The strategy of translation has some decided advantages and disadvantages. First, translation is a metaphor that grants each of the various language systems its own integrity and separateness. As such it is a safeguard against baptizing a specific language as Christian: Christian behaviorism, Christian phenomenology, Christian psychoanalysis, or Christian family systems therapy. Second, the language metaphor makes relative all languages, which then frees the individual Christian professional to use a variety of languages. This means that the language of contemporary Christianity is not made absolute either. Integration of Christianity and psychotherapy is not simply a return to the exclusive use of biblical language; therapy is not simply chanting Bible verses. No one language has a corner on reality. Furthermore, one can use one language to counter the biases of others. Phenomenologically oriented psychological theories are a good counter for more empirically oriented approaches.

This strategy also has some besetting weaknesses. First, the language or theory into which the story of the Reign of God is translated tends to take on primacy and "givenness." This seems for me to be the case in some of the examples provided above. When this happens, the vision of Christianity is rewritten in the language of the prevailing (therapeutic) culture. One wonders whether in principle the Christian should not avoid commitment to any one psychological approach. One can be eclectic, use many languages, and thus reduce the possibility of equating Christianity with only one translation. Second, it is easy for us to assume that a particular translation (even if it is eclectic) is permanent. Translation changes as external circumstances change. Reification of a translation too easily raises the translation to the level of dogma. Such an approach is too static. Third, languages are not entirely neutral. They do reflect implicit assumptions about the nature of reality; they become metaphysical. They do not remain simply descriptive but begin to extrapolate arbitrarily about the nature and purpose of life, ultimate values, and the nature of God. Nevertheless, cleared of their presumed normativity, a variety of languages are clearly useful to the Christian professional. Fourth, this strategy easily forgets that something always "falls between the cracks" in the process of translation. Christianity comes to us in a language embodied in culture. The test of the adequacy of the translation must be the faithfulness to the praxis of the New Testament church.

Critical to this strategy is the context in which the translation takes place since translators often work entirely alone and then submit their work as final. For the Christian, in whatever occupation, that context is the church. Here the essential dimensions of the vision are hammered out and the translation tested for adequacy. Translation should be a fundamentally communal process.

Dialogue

The Strategy

The relationship of church and profession in this fourth metaphor for the church/profession relationship is one of dialogue. It is a dialogue of tension and paradox: Christ and culture in terms of the relationship of God's righteousness versus human righteousness. Our relationship to God is a relationship that has been broken by sin and has been reconciled through the death of Christ. The conflict between God and humankind is viewed from the perspective of God's grace and human sin; a recognition of this state does not change the nature of the situation: conflict remains. Grace is unconditional; sin is radical. Before the holiness of God, all human works are corrupt, regardless of whether they are performed within the church or without. Christ's law applies to all persons, not simply those who are spiritual giants. Culture embodies the human lust for power. It is only God's grace that sustains us in the midst of this morass. The relationship between Christ and culture is then one of tension and paradox. We function simultaneously under law that condemns and grace that forgives. We speak of revelation and use reason, view Christ as Creator and Redeemer, and see humankind as both sinful and justified.

Niebuhr (1951) finds Luther the best representative of this motif. Luther wrote and thought in a time of national and religious turmoil. For him, there were two reigns: the Reign of God and that of this world. The first deals with the moral life and sets persons free to work in the world of culture. One develops the spirit of humanity, the other focuses on technique. The relationship of Christ and culture for Luther is dynamic and dialectical.

Niebuhr's assessment of this position states that it reflects accurately the life of the Christian who lives between the times. "It is a report of an experience rather than a plan or campaign" (165). Further, this position is more sensitive to the dynamic interaction of God and the person, between sin and grace. Humanity responds to God's action toward us. It has also provided new resolution for commitment, and emancipation from custom and tradition that have usurped the Living Lord.

Application

My proposal is to grant that at times the relationship between church and profession is a dialogue between two very separate entities, but that both are significant partners in the dialogue. The metaphor of conversation as a way of describing the relationship of church and profession is appropriate in view of the finiteness of our expressions of faith and also the finiteness of cultural achievements. It recognizes that all theological constructions are human constructions bound to a greater or lesser extent by the social, historical, psychological, and economic conditions in which we live. The same can, of course, be said of the professional achievements. It is a stance, then, of partners in dialogue.

In genuine dialogue both partners in the conversation are changed as a result of the interaction. For such dialogue to occur it is appropriate for both members to bracket their preconceived notions, to listen empathically to the other, and to set aside any demands one might have of the other. Furthermore, one must expect that the other also has something significant to contribute. It is a creative encounter in which the unexpected is a possibility, disagreement is accepted, and tension welcomed rather than avoided. It recognizes the uniqueness the other brings to the conversation as a result of a different history of experiences. Genuine dialogue requires the energy necessary to reconstruct the perspective of another. The further apart the reference groups that have shaped our particular constellation of attitudes and our construction of reality, the greater the differences partners bring to the encounter. But "respons-ability" implies responsibility to engage in dialogue.

What then can we learn from a dialogue with the social sciences? From Freud we can learn that religion is sometimes projection, a satisfaction of individual wishes (Freud, 1927/1961, 1936/1961; Kueng, 1979). Freud would have said it in a less qualified way. Nonetheless, greater honesty about one's own motivation is appropriate. Also, Freud's sensitivity to the effects of an oppressive society on the individual (sexually or otherwise) needs to be heard. He detailed the havoc created, the fragmentation of the self, and the guilt that comes with an oversocialized superego. Jung has reminded us of the importance of tradition and symbol in the life of the individual, even though Jung accepts the myths of culture in a rather democratic manner as the foundation of the modern individual (Jung, 1933). Skinner (1971) is right when he argues that we are conditioned. We do well to examine the ways in which this occurs in American society. However, Skinner can be criticized for overstepping the bounds of objective research when he argues for the essential meaninglessness of human freedom simply because we cannot find examples of where we are not conditioned. Erikson (1953) has described child development in Western societies in a helpful way. He has shown how a technological and capitalistic society has shaped the process of growth, though he was less sensitive to the effects of sexism.

The advantage of this metaphor of dialogue is its willingness to accept tension and to live with it. A problem implicit in the position is that, in spite of the emphasis on dialogue, compartmentalization results when it is assumed that each member in the conversation is bound by roles: Clinicians are to deal with emotional issues while pastors are responsible for bringing religious insights to bear on therapy. Such a dichotomy will only serve to rationalize the status quo.

Witness

The Strategy

Niebuhr (1951) refers to this approach as conversionist. It accepts Christ's judgment of culture but refers to Christ the redeemer rather than the giver of the new law. He deals with what is deepest in humanity, not the external. The self-destructiveness of humanity and culture lies in its self-contradictoriness. Yet culture is under God's sovereign rule, and cultural work must be carried out in obedience to Christ. Creation is not sacrificed to redemption. "All things were created, in heaven and on earth, visible, and invisible, whether thrones or dominions, or principalities or authorities—all things were created through him and for him" (Col. 1:16). The creative activity of God is a major theme. Christ is seen in both his incarnation and his death. Sin in culture is seen as perversion rather than as ontological evil. "The problem of culture is therefore the problem of its conversion, not of its replacement by a new creation; though the conversion is so radical that it amounts to a kind of rebirth" (1951:194). History is viewed not simply as a consequence of human acts but always as a dramatic interaction between God and humankind. It is the story of God's mighty deeds and humanity's response to them. The focus is on the present transformation by the Lord of all things cultural for the glory of God.

Niebuhr sees this theme running through the fourth gospel. For John, whatever is, is good given the incarnation of the Word (John 1:1). Sin is a denial of the principle of life itself. Niebuhr states:

> It can only be said that in general John's interest is directed toward the spiritual transformation of man's life in the world, not toward the substitution of a wholly spiritual existence for a temporal one, nor toward the replacement of the present physical environment and bodies of men by new physical and metaphysical creations, nor toward the gradual ascent from the temporal to the eternal (1951:204).

In Augustine, Niebuhr suggests, we have a clear illustration of this model of Christ/culture relationship. Augustine expects a universal regeneration through Christ. Augustine illustrates in his own life the transformation of culture, as one who has been converted from being pagan to becoming Christian. He uses language with a new brilliance. While he uses the neo-Platonism of the time, it is given new depth and direction; it is humanized. The result is medieval Christendom. As the trans-former of culture, Augustine redirects, reinvigorates, and regenerates human works that in present reality are perverted, but were created good. Calvin follows the same motif in his call for the permeation of all of life with the Gospel. Vocations express faith and we may glorify God in our callings.

Application

I will reconstruct Niebuhr's description of this strategy as *witness*. In this strategy for the application of the Church-culture relationship to psychology, the focus is on the distinctive contribution of the church. By providing a different context for cultural achievements, something new is created that clearly reflects the Judeo-Christian heritage. It takes seriously the assumption that there is a uniquely Christian way of viewing some issues. It assumes that we begin with the fact of God's existence in our understanding of human nature, healing, and society. It views history as the arena of God's activity that began with the mighty deeds recorded by the Israelites and the New Testament Christians, and that continues today. Our par-ticipation in that history, our work and purposes, are then understood and judged most clearly from the perspective of Yahweh. All of life is to be permeated with the Gospel. Christ is the redeemer of the world. The style of this strategy is a call for change in conformity with the fundamental vision of the Reign of God.

There are some distinct beliefs that emerge out of my Believers' Church heritage that have implications for our approaches in mental health practice. While there may be no coherent Believers' Church position from which to build a model of therapy, there are distinct individual themes that can be fruitfully explored. The following directions might be pursued.

1. *Pluralism.* It is entirely inconsistent to engage in theo-logical imperialism in therapy when, historically, indi-viduals in the Believers' Churches died for religious pluralism (e.g., the Anabaptists). Religious liberty allows us to exercise and explore the implications of

our faith stance. That same freedom guarantees the freedom of the clients not to believe the way a therapist does and not to be rejected or turned away because of it. Religious pluralism grants integrity to the person who is not a Christian. That independence is also respected even when the therapist or mental health program points to an alternative way of life. Pluralism assumes that people are at different stages in their attitude toward the kingdom of God. That allows for the possibility that even in therapy a counselor may make explicit reference to faith dimensions without imperialism.

2. *Voluntarism.* Pluralism grants a person the right to choose; voluntarism assumes the person has the ability to choose. If it is assumed that the image of God in us is not so completely obliterated by sin that a moral response is impossible, then the individual can be held accountable. Where there is no ability to respond, accountability is not the issue. Where clinical judgment indicates that the individual is capable of choosing, accepting the consequences of action, and being self-aware to a greater degree, therapeutic strategies would also change and expectations would be greater.

3. *Discipleship.* Much of contemporary therapy has focused on gospel to the exclusion of law. Such a separation is problematic in theology and in therapy. It results in acceptance without confrontation, individual actualization instead of sacrifice, and freedom without structure. Discipleship assumes that the model set by Christ is what it means to be human. Here there is no dichotomy between gospel and law. Whether the client is a Christian or not, to the extent that one's life is patterned on this model, new life is a possibility. This does not assume that there is one ethic for Christians and another for those who choose not to be. For the therapist there is only one ethic, though different individuals bring different resources to the encounter.

4. *Covenant.* Life is not lived alone nor is life understood only from an individual perspective. God's covenant with the human race remains unbroken and, hence, human life can be understood only in the light of that

covenant—and covenant language applies also to human relationships. To live a life of discipleship in secret was impossible for Anabaptists. Covenant characterized all of life. Therapy would then include restoration of covenant both with God and humanity.

5. Priesthood of all believers. Before God we are all priests. No distinction is made between clergy and laity. All are called to minister to the needs of brother, sister, and neighbor. The church then would be a significant context for healing. We have a long way to go in recognizing the Christian community as a resource for healing the broken. At least part of the problem is that the present nature and structure of the church precludes it. One can effect little change when "church" means meeting Sunday morning and Wednesday night. But in the context of small covenant groups that take seriously each other's welfare, healing is possible. The therapist then functions less as an individual and more in conjunction with a specific community.

The church is caught between the temptations of assimilation and isolation. In terms of the strategies listed above, assimilation occurs most easily when we are defensive about a critique, obsess on continuity, assume the identity of languages, underestimate the differences between the partners in dialogue, and minimize the uniqueness of the Christian contribution. On the other hand, isolation is a consequence of exclusive critique, rejection of all continuity, widening the differences between languages, compartmentalizing the partners in the dialogue, and proclaiming imperialistically the church's distinctiveness. None of these modes of response is acceptable.

Part 3

The Therapist as Ethical Character

8

On Character

From a systems perspective it is appropriate to assume that all that has been said of larger systems (culture and community) is applicable to the smaller subsystems—the individual (Gergen, 1991). But what is the nature of the connection? It is in the nature of religion to be integrative, and so I seek consistency and harmony between the various foci: cultural, communal, and individual. But I seek more than mere logical consistency, I hope for a consistency of ethical vision. Thus the story of the Reign of God and the discerned ethic and praxis of the Christian community form the character and the virtues of the healer (Smith, 1981). Where there is inconsistency, the possibility of healing and effectiveness is reduced. The story of the Reign of God calls for peace, justice, mercy, and faithfulness. When the Christian community embodies in some measure that story, the possibility increases that healers emerge whose character and therapeutic efforts reflect those values.

This section will attempt to bring forward the concerns of the previous sections and focus them on the individual therapist. Character and healing are inextricably intertwined. The therapist with character that reflects the Reign of God is sensitive to sociopolitical contexts and the role of culture in therapy. Such a therapist recognizes that therapy is an ethical process. The therapist sensitive to the church as a community of ethical dis-

173

cernment sees his or her work as a gift, qualifies the authority of the professional community, and rejects individualism.

This third section will examine the individual therapist's character, a narrower focus than that of culture and community (see Dykstra, 1981; Gustafson, 1968; Niebuhr, 1963; Hallie, 1979; Malony, 1983). The first chapter reflects on the nature of character from an ethical perspective. The second chapter will explore the meaning of the ethical language of character within modernity. The third chapter will delineate an alternate model for personal development of therapists. I will conclude with a description of and reflections on my own experiences while traveling between Jerusalem and Athens.

One healer of whom it can be said that narrative, community, and character are integrated is Mother Theresa (Le Joly, 1983). Her life reflects the ethic of the larger Christian story and the praxis of a specific ethical community. Although Mother Theresa's work might not be considered psychotherapy or counseling in the modern Western sense, it is certainly healing in its desire to bring people, particularly the poor, toward wholeness and health.

In 1946 Mother Theresa felt called to leave her convent and help the poor of India while living among them. She did that, establishing a new order that would minister to the needs of the poorest of the poor. Since that time she has opened homes for the destitute, taking in people who would have died alone on the streets. She has begun orphanages, homes for the handicapped and the abandoned, schools for children, and shelters for the leprous. In various other ways she has met the physical and spiritual, social and emotional needs of the very poor.

In many ways Mother Teresa illustrates the faithful healer who is virtuous because of her ethical culture, community, and character. The story of the Reign of God makes it possible to find meaning in suffering and a posture of powerlessness. The Sisters of Charity are for her an ethical community of praxis. These provide a context for and coherence to her work. But more, her character reflects this story and practice. Her way of life is self-sacrificial and full of joy. The lifetime covenant that she has made shapes the nature of her character. Her vows can be summarized as obedience, poverty, chastity, and free service to the poor. The Western model of fee-for-service, professional accreditation, and self-actualization is irrelevant.

Can one argue with integrity that the character of the therapist is irrelevant to the healing process? Imagine a therapist who lives the life of a philanderer outside of therapy but assumes that his or her counseling is not affected. Consider a psychologist who is unconcerned about sociopolitical issues, who is never engaged in the active search for gender sensitivity and the responsible use of environmental resources. Can this same psychologist also assume that these larger contextual issues are irrelevant to the psychotherapeutic process?

In this section I will argue the contrary. I do not think life can be so compartmentalized without a price to be paid. As with Mother Theresa, the character of the healer may well affect the quality of the healing. Character is not incidental to the effectiveness of healing. Mother Theresa sees character as developed, not inherent. Ritual is ubiquitous in her life. She trains herself and her sisters through education, worship, and practice. She supervises them to maintain consistency with the Christian story and the specific convictions of their community. She advises, "I do not want you to perform miracles with unkindness; rather, I prefer you to make mistakes in kindness" (Le Joly, 1983:59). It shows.

I will begin this chapter with a discussion of the self as ethical, using the work of rabbi Heschel (1965) as a foundation. Then a more careful analysis of the meaning of character in terms of story, convictions, and virtue will be given. I will propose that two metaphors (covenant-maker and reconciler) and two virtues (faithfulness and powerlessness) are of critical importance to the character of the healer who takes the Reign of God as frame of reference.

Human Nature as Ethical

The central thesis of this section is reflected in Abraham Heschel's Stanford lectures (1965). He makes a distinction between "human being" and "being human." To focus on human being is to assume that the critical anthropological question is "What is the human being?" and that the appropriate answer is that the individual is one of many manifestations of being. Being human, on the other hand, suggests that the only acceptable answer is that the individual is a living person of whom ethical demands are made. Metaphysically, the first perspective is oriented toward ontology, while the second is existential-ethical. Epistemologically, the focus on the person as an aspect of being moves toward knowledge as descriptive information of the individual as an object in time and space. The emphasis on being human points to knowledge as meaning that involves knowing how to live (wisdom). Those, in broad strokes, are the differences.

Human Being

To say that a person is human being is to say that what is human can be derived from the category of being. What then is the nature of being? What is its structure? From Heschel's perspective, being is the brute facticity of existence in time and space. It is patterned, regular, repetitive, and continuous. As such it is measurable, manipulable, and predictable. Human being is an extension of being. In Heschel's words: "Human being shares the being of all beings, just as champagne and shoe polish, cheesecake and pebbles" (96). Both human beings and animals have basic needs and desires that need to be satisfied. In many ways both are reactive to the natural and social environment. Development is then similar to the evolution of all species of being. That which is distinctive of human being emerges from a comparison with other levels of being.

Knowledge of the human being, in Heschel's view, is fragmented because the many perspectives of the person as object cannot be integrated. As object, the individual can be measured, counted, analyzed, and averaged. The knowledge that is produced is best referred to as information. The major assumption is that the structure of being is comprehensible by reason and the human being is then explicable as a part of a larger taxonomy of being. Truth is the correspondence of an idea with the structure of being. The knowledge obtained is used to manipulate the world of things and people. "Oughtness," in this paradigm, is derived from the nature of that which *is*, namely, being.

Being Human

Being human is the experience of life as an ethical problem. It is the experience of contradiction between existence and expectation. Rather than being a consequence of curiosity, being human is the embarrassment of knowing too much (the difference between what is and what ought to be), and the embarrassment of living in the presence of the divine and not knowing it.

Being human always involves an ethic of meaning. Meaning assumes that there is a larger context of existence that provides a sense of order. That larger context is a transcendent context and is not a theoretical system or set of universal laws. Meaning emerges from conscious acts. There is no meaning in what one is, only in what one does. Meaning is not the satisfaction of personal needs, but is found in the satisfaction of the needs of others. Meaning emerges out of our response to the God who seeks us. The Greeks, according to Heschel, saw meaning as a search for an idea, whereas the Jews saw it as God in search of humanity. Meaning is, then, dependent on response. The meaning of being human is concurring with God's vision of our task.

Being human is mystery. The person is not explicable in the same way as is an object in time and space. When rationality is primary, that which is inexplicable is irrational. Mystery is not a synonym for the unknown, but rather, a term for meaning that stands in relation to Mystery. The mystery of the "I am" evokes wonder and awe.

Being human means appreciation, not manipulation. Manipulation sees humans as objects and information, as means to an end. It leads to alienation and the death of transcendence. It's supreme value is expediency. Appreciation, however, sees the world in terms of acknowledgment and understanding. It leads to fellowship and the affirmation of the possibilities of life. It recognizes that, while we are called to master the earth, we did not create it.

Being human is living. The deed is the distillation of the self. Sheer being, however, is passive, anonymous, and intransitive. In living, the person relates actively to the world in deeds. Living is giving form to being. Being human is an act, and hence, the opposite of being is not nonbeing but what is done with personal being.

Being human means being responsible. Adam's first encounter with Yahweh is a command to care for the land and to populate it. Yahweh's response to nature is the commandment of creation. Philosophically, the primacy of creation over being means that the "ought" precedes "is." The order of things goes back to an "order" of God. Obedience is the response to the primacy of ought. "Thou art" precedes "I am." "I am because I am called upon to be." Heschel states, "What I suggest is not that first there is neutral being and then values. Being created implies being born in value, being endowed with meaning and receiving value. Living involves acceptance of meaning, obedience, commitment" (1965:98).

Character as Metaphor

One of the ways healing is mediated is through the character of the healer. From Heschel's view of being human, a therapist can be considered an ethical agent, a sacral individual. In classical societies, Greco-Roman and Judeo-Christian, the healer is assumed to be an exemplary figure, one whose life reflects the ideals of the culture. MacIntyre (1981) has therefore suggested that characters are "the moral representatives of their culture and they are so because of the way in which moral and metaphysical ideas and theories assume through them an embodied existence in the social world. Characters are the masks worn by moral philosophies" (1981:27). The notion of character is treated with regard by a culture because the character furnishes us with a cultural and moral ideal. Character legitimates a mode of existence. MacIntyre chooses the term "character" because it combines dramatic and moral associations, story, and ethics.

Sacral character is shaped by a unique story considered normative and by convictions communally discerned. The result is character that is made coherent around specific metaphors and particular virtues that embody the story and the convictions in personal action. To talk of the therapist's character assumes that the goodness of persons is not automatic but cultivated. It is created through the routine of ritual.

First let me reflect more generally on the nature of character. To speak of character is to refer to what is deliberative, purposive, and behavioral. Character, I assume, is reflected in a coherence of behavioral acts and consistency in motivation. What the theme of story can do at the cultural level and discernment at the communal level, I hope character can do at the personal level. Character is not simply an assemblage of personality traits. It is what makes one predictable and consistent. To have character, suggests James McLendon (1974), is to enter at a new level the realm of morality, the level at which one's person, with its continuities, its interconnections, its integrity, is intimately involved in one's deeds. By being the person we are, we are able to do what we do and conversely, by those very deeds we form or re-form our own characters. . . . Thus character is paradoxically both the cause and consequence of what we do (30–31).

Character provides a way of making concrete the normative nature of the Christian life. It involves what we have traditionally called the process of sanctification. Hauerwas's definition of character is that

on a theological level, the idea of a character provides a way of explicating the normative nature of the Christian life. The Christian life is not simply a matter of assuming a vague loving attitude, but rather it is a concrete determination of our being developed through our history. . . . This formation is the determination of our character through God's sanctifying work. Sanctification is thus the formation of the Christian's character that is the result of his intention to see the world as redeemed in Jesus Christ (1974:67).

Character is related to story, convictions, and virtues. I will examine each in turn.

Story

As previously stated, the primary story that serves as context for the Christian healer is the story of the Reign of God. That story is not abstract. It consists of particular persons, events, and ideas. The individual healer is one whose memory is marked by the events of the Christian story of Yahweh's interaction with humanity. The image of disciple in that story points to one who seeks to embody the ethic of the Reign of God. Again, Hauerwas:

To be agents at all requires a directionality. Such attention is formed and given content by the stories through which we have learned to form the story of our lives. To be moral persons is to allow stories to be told through us so that our manifold activities gain a coherence that allows us to claim them for our own. The significance of stories is the significance of character for the moral life as our experience itself, if it is to be coherent, is but an incipient story (1974:26).

Convictions

Religious communities seek to nurture a practical and convictional faith in their members. Character is shaped by convictions, by particular ways of seeing and being in the world. Convictions are integral to faith. They are the tenaciously held beliefs that give definiteness to the personality of an individual or community. If they are surrendered, the individual is profoundly changed. Convictions are not simply abstract principles. They are more concrete. Convictions emerge out of the stories (worldview and ethos) of particular communities. With their intentions, individuals express bodies of moral belief in their action. Intentions presume bodies of belief. The actions and convictions of the disciple are intelligible against a larger scheme of beliefs.

Virtue

The sacral healer is one whose character is defined by specific behavioral virtues consistent with the ideals of the body politic. For the follower of Christ those virtues are consistent with the Christian story and the discernment of the Christian community. MacIntyre (1981) has pointed out that classical cultures possessed a conceptual scheme that indicated what is required by a given social role inhabited by an individual; a conception of excellences or virtues as those qualities that enable an individual to do what his or her role requires; and a conception of the human condition as fragile and vulnerable. Hauerwas states:

> We are as we come to see and as that seeing becomes enduring in our intentionality. We do not come to see, however, just by looking but by training our vision through the metaphors and symbols that constitute our central convictions. How we come to see therefore is a function of how we come to be since our seeing necessarily is determined by how our basic images are embodied by the self—i.e., in our character. Christian ethics is the conceptual discipline that analyzes and imaginatively tests the images most appropriate to score the Christian life in accordance with the central conviction that the world has been

redeemed by the work and person of Christ (1974:2).

Metaphors for the Character of the Therapist

What critical qualities of the healer's character are consistent with the Christian story? In lieu of the image of the self-sufficient, rational, and expert professional, we would like to explore two biblical images that run counter to the therapeutic culture: the Christian as covenant-maker and as reconciler. Righteousness is central to each of them.

Covenant-Maker

Much has been made of the importance of contractual relationships between therapist and client. We would submit that contract is the very least we can do, but it is hardly adequate as a metaphor to shape character or the therapeutic process. In his fascinating article entitled "Covenanting as Human Vocation," Walter Breuggemann (1979) makes an articulate case for the following thesis: "Covenant is the dominant metaphor for Biblical faith by which human personality can be understood" (13). It should be noted immediately that Brueggemann thinks of covenanting as *metaphor,* not dogma. This is consistent with our assumption that character is shaped by images and metaphors. The metaphor of covenant points to the fact that human persons "are grounded in Another who initiates personhood and who stays bound to persons in loyal ways for their well being" (14). Such a view of the self, of course, contradicts any attempt at self-groundedness. Brueggeman's definition of covenant assumes that the God of the Old and New Testament is one who wills, keeps, and makes covenants. That would suggest that one of the marks of the Christian healer is his or her ability to develop and maintain covenants in marriage, friendship, or therapy.

Brueggemann describes the covenant-making God as one who has the power to make something new. This is in sharp contrast to deterministic and naturalistic psychological ideologies. The covenant-making God makes something new through speech. By God's word the earth is created; it is creative speech. Covenant making involves speech. So also does therapy. The covenant-making therapist is one who does so in the image of a covenant-making God. Further, the covenant-mak-

ing God is one who holds on to the covenant partner so that the
life of the partner is ordained to deal with God. Brueggemann
points out that the specific form of this holding of the covenant
partner to God is Torah—i.e., the gift of guidance and suste-
nance. The covenant-making healer is one who views the troubled individual as one called to deal with God.

Brueggemann then goes on to describe the appropriate
responses of a covenant partnership to the covenant-making
God. A faithful human response is hope. It is the confidence of
the healer that Yahweh will be faithful to our clients. Second,
faithful human action is to listen as the covenant-making God
speaks. Israel is continually indicted for not listening (Jer.
5:21; 7:13; 11:10; 13:11). The covenant-keeping healer is, above
all, one capable of listening. Third, Brueggemann suggests that
faithful human action involves obedient answering language.
Such obedience manifests itself in the doing of justice and
righteousness, of being loyal and gracious. At issue here is not
self-actualization or self-discovery by the healer but a life lived
righteously.

Fourth, Brueggemann argues that faithful human action in
the face of a covenant-making God is to rage and protest
against the condition of human civilization. Indeed, it is an act
of arrogance to assume that the human condition is our responsibility alone. The Old Testament believer held Yahweh
accountable as covenant-partner to redeem the world. So also
the Christian healer is one who mediates healing by holding
Yahweh responsible for the healing. Fifth, it is faithful human
action in the presence of a covenant-making God to grieve, and
finally, to praise the giver of all gifts. Brueggemann points out
that the practices of grief, rage, and praise make possible the
posture of hope, listening, and answering. The first triad is
clearly dramatic, liturgical, and public. The covenantal healer
is one who is deeply immersed in such ritual that, in turn,
shapes character. He states that "it is the faithful doing of conventional actions that makes covenantal life possible" (15).

Brueggemann suggests that this model of covenanting as
human vocation has the following implications. It transposes
all identity questions into vocational questions. At issue is not
self-focused self-definition, but rather, an identity that is given
in the call of the One. Identity emerges in the interaction
between the One who calls and the one who is called. The

agenda between the two is a calling. The Christian's calling is to covenanting, to faithfulness, and to service in the world. A second implication of a covenantal view of the self is that personal existence is then, by definition, conflicted. There is a tension between what we are and what it is we are called to be. What is promised in the covenant relationship is not equilibrium or even wholeness but God's faithfulness to us in the midst of contradiction. The metaphor of covenant-maker is a rich one for the therapist in comparison with contract metaphors. This will require the reevaluation of the other dominant metaphors in Western society: professional clinician and pragmatist. A conventional theology assumes that the ethical stance of the therapist is not simply a personal position. The therapist who is Christian seeks to embody the covenantal righteousness of Christ and to model for the client appropriate responses to stresses in the life cycle.

Reconciler

It might be argued that in Paul we have an example of character that is healing. Indeed, I would argue that Paul is principally a reconciler and that this is another critical metaphor for contemporary therapists. Like the metaphor of covenant, it tends to move one away from a simplistic preoccupation with an intrapsychic agenda. The apostle Paul is often seen as an individual at peace with himself because he experiences no guilt. He has a conversion experience and is "born again." He has experienced forgiveness and lives with a clear conscience. He is justified before God by faith, not works. He lives without guilt. His life is whole and purposeful. Certainly such a character is a prerequisite for mediating healing.

In 1961, Krister Stendahl delivered an invited address to the annual meeting of the American Psychological Association (of all places). It was entitled "The Apostle Paul and the Introspective Conscience of the West." In this article (and later a book that expands his thesis), he proposes that we have fundamentally misread the apostle Paul. We have hailed him as the hero of introspective consciousness with the text: "I do not do the good I want, but the evil I do not want to do is what I do" (Rom. 7:19). He argues that we have projected the troubled conscience of the West on Paul on the presupposition that humanity basically remains the same throughout all ages. This line of reasoning then suggests that Paul's experience of justification by faith is the resolution of his guilt. Stendahl argues that this view of Paul is rooted in Augustine, the piety of the Middle Ages, and Luther's struggle with his own conscience. But it was not Paul's agenda.

We have tended to read Paul on this issue in terms of the grounds or terms by which we are to be saved. Stendahl's argument is that in the book of Romans, "Paul's focus really is the relation between Jews and Gentiles, not the notion of justification or predestination and certainly not other proper yet abstract theological topics" (1976:4). What we have done is to take Paul's experience with the Gentiles and make it a timeless commentary on the nature of faith. Stendahl suggests that the early church seems to have felt that Paul spoke about what he actually spoke about, the reconciliation of Jews and Gentiles.

The character of the Christian therapist is one who seeks for and prays for reconciliation between people, between neurotic mother and victimized son, between estranged daughter and alienated parents, between feuding families, between spouses living in separate worlds, between rich and poor, male and female, master and slave. Stendahl suggests that one reason we focus on personal forgiveness is because we

> possess a strong psychological bent and there is no question that the term in any quest for relief from sin and guilt which works best within a psychological framework is "forgiveness." What makes this sort of quest so central—and again I guess—is that it is related to the fact that we happen to be more interested in ourselves than in God or in the fate of his creation (18).

The Therapist and Critical Christian Virtues

From this discussion of primary metaphors for the character of the Christian healer, we move on now to suggest that there are some critical virtues in the character of the Christian healer: faithfulness and powerlessness.

Faithfulness

Lebacqz (1985) suggests that the primary virtue of professionals is that of independent trusteeship. They are carriers of the cultural tradition of a society or an alternative society. The healer is one who carries the memory and who articulates its perspective. To be a trustee means to be trustworthy, trusted, faithful. This is consistent with the fact that the God we serve is one who maintains faithfulness to covenant—that is, steadfast love. Thus, if the Christian therapist symbolizes God's covenant and redeeming activity toward humankind, this means even a greater stress on being trustworthy. This is central to the Christian story. To violate trust is not simply to be unprofessional, but also to undermine the story of Yahweh as faithful.

To be faithful, behaviorally and therapeutically, is to assume that there is no guarantee of healing but that we will seek to remain faithful and present to a counselee. Faithfulness in the therapist will manifest itself in one's relationship to one's spouse, to one's church, and to our God. In terms of therapy, to heal the chronically ill is to be faithful to them by creating a setting in which there is safety and the opportunity for growth. To be faithful to the poor is to be accessible, and to adapt one's therapeutic approach. To be faithful may on occasion be more important than effectiveness.

Powerlessness

Lebacqz (1985) stresses that an image that needs renewal among professionals is that of the suffering servant who is characterized by the willingness to absorb someone else's pain. Therapeutic hope is the ability, in spite of a client's loss of hope, to maintain hope. It is by Christ's stripes that we are healed. Thereby, the negative has been deprived of its ultimacy.

Lebacqz feels that the suffering servant image is particularly important in response to the issue of power in professionalism. Guggenbuehl-Craig (1986) has described the exercise of power by the therapist over the client. This may be done blatantly when the client's value system is clearly different from that of the professional, but the professional has the social sanction to demand change (separation, placement, hospitalization, or other action). The power drive is given its freest expression when it can appear under the cloak of objectivity, moral rectitude, and competence. This is aggravated when one assumes the role of the omniscient professional.

Modern modes of healing tend to separate character and virtue from healing. Somehow the concrete, embodied historical life of the healer has become less relevant to the therapeutic process. The ethical images of covenant-maker and reconciler are, I think, critical in the development of the cultured therapist. The character of those who call themselves Christians may then begin to reflect their normative culture and community.

9

Enlightenment
Morality Redux

Therapists are, after all, subject to the same destructive forces as their clients. They are not simply immunized technicians. It is highly conceivable then that the healer may suffer from the same malady as those in need of healing. It is important that we reflect on the extent to which the role played, the life lived, and the vision hoped for by the clinical psychologist who is a Christian reflects the ethos of the Christian community. Our era will need therapists whose character is transformed to see the needs of the poor, the neglected, and the emotionally troubled regardless of race, gender, religion, or social class. Both religious and professional communities are concerned about the apparent loss of ethical sensibilities.

We have well-articulated ethical regulations but lack the moral ethos to sustain them. Pope, Tabachnick, and Keith-Spiegel (1987) have reported extensively on the ethical practices of psychologists. They report that number one in the ten greatest causes of successful cases against psychologists from 1976–1986 was sexual contact (18.5 percent). There is considerable concern expressed within the therapeutic community about whether there are not more violations than those reported, and whether a profession as a community is able to sustain the ethical behavior of its members.

Hence, standard textbooks on ethics in therapy (Corey, Corey, and Callanan, 1984; Keith-Spiegel and Koocher 1985; Kottler and Van Hoose, 1977) usually examine both ethical decision making and the personality of the therapist. The texts review the ethical issues of confidentiality, value imposition, abuse reporting, competence, therapist-client relationships, etc. Corey, Corey, and Callanan (1984) also describe the critical personality variabilities of the ethical therapist. They list nine: good will, the ability to be present for others, willingness to be vulnerable and take risks, self-respect and self-appreciation, willingness to serve as models, willingness to risk making mistakes, and a growth orientation. They go on to include the willingness of the therapist to bracket personal needs and unresolved personal conflicts for the sake of the client. Therapists should have no need to control the client or depend on the client's approval. Compulsive advice giving and an obsessive need to develop social relationships with clients should be dealt with. In other words, countertransference tendencies are capable of resolution.

In this chapter I will reflect on the nature of character in modern perspective. I begin with a summary of various forces shaping the discussion of character. Thereafter I will focus on one theory of moral development, its implications for therapists, and conclude with some critical reflections.

Forces Shaping the Discussion of Character

If a critique of modern culture and an ethical evaluation of healing were to point to the destructive effects on the therapeutic process of all the "isms"—pluralism, secularism, capitalism, individualism, pragmatism, sexism, racism, or ageism—what would be our response in terms of how character is conceived? Would we continue to train therapists in the current scientist-practitioner model of healing? It is not accessible to the poor. The mechanisms of accountability are weak. If the healing is biased against women or the poor, who would know (Hare-Mustin, 1978, 1987)? It makes little use of community resources beyond the session itself. The scientist-practitioner model tends to separate character from technique. Somehow the concrete, embodied historical life of the healer becomes irrelevant to the therapeutic process.

Western Culture

The ethical confusion and pragmatism of Western culture militates against a serious consideration of the nature and importance of the character of healers. As stated earlier, the moral languages of contemporary Western culture are fragmented and incoherent. Consensus about the nature of good character has become virtually impossible, except perhaps in some coherent subcultures. The nature of the particular character of an agent of healing is, then, also in question. Further, the development of therapists as ethical agents is hindered by the fact that a technological culture tends to produce healers unable to engage in ethical reflection. MacIntye (1981) suggests that modern culture has produced therapists who see ends as beyond the scope of change. We are unable to enter into moral debate because we restrict ourselves to the realm of fact, means, and measurable effectiveness.

The Analytic Attitude

In his most significant book, *The Triumph of the Therapeutic,* Phillip Rieff (1966) makes a distinction between two types of therapy. The relevance for the discussion here is that the importance of the character of the therapist is different in each of the models. Based on his research on Freud, Rieff delineates two therapeutic traditions: analytic and commitment.

Analytic therapies emerge in the modern, postindustrial world of democratic individualism and are designed to meet the needs of the communally detached individual. This model of therapy, based primarily on the work of Freud, makes no claim that well-being is dependent on membership in a political community. It tends to assume the fundamental sufficiency of the self. The purpose of therapy tends toward separation and individuation from community in order for well-being to occur. The individual must free the self from binding attachments to communities in order to express one's individuality. The analytic therapist, personally, has no normative community that he/she represents. Freud did not posit a well-differentiated, constructive social theory. Analytic therapies are informative; they provide the patient with information that was not personally available. In analytic therapies the counselor is not expected to be sacral or exemplary, only to be skilled analytically. Indeed, one is to be more anonymous in order to allow transference to occur. In the analytic therapies any techniques that work are used since there are few external, communal restrictions considered normative.

Commitment therapies are more common in minority and non-Western cultures. They assume that, ultimately, it is communities that cure. In commitment therapy the function is to commit the patient to the symbol system of the therapist's community, and well-being is defined as the development of a collective identity. The commitment therapist cures by reinforcing the best in the cultural superego. The community is assumed to be salvific. Salvation is defined as an experience that transforms all personal relations by subordinating them to communal purposes.

Behind the traditionalist commitment therapist, whether shaman or priest, stands culture as healer. The healer speaks for the corporate identity. Commitment therapies are transformative; they assume that a transformation of the self is necessary in order to enter or reenter the community. The therapist is considered a sacral figure who is exemplary in that his or her life reflects the ideals of the culture or community. The therapist, in commitment therapies, is permitted to use the salvific stories, images, artifacts, or rituals of the community because of the trust that has been conferred. The techniques used are those sanctioned by the community.

The assumptions regarding the importance and substance of character are very different in each of the models of therapy. In analytic approaches character is limited primarily to technique. In the commitment therapies character follows in substance the cultural ideals the therapist represents. One takes too seriously the individual, while the other absolutizes culture.

Self-Fulfillment Ideology

Self-realization, it is asserted, is a function of introspection, clarification of personal values, and creating balance between opposing forces. It is assumed that the individual is self-sufficient, that introspection is the road to personal development, and that freedom is the critical moral value. For Jung, the characterological ideal is the individual profoundly sensitive to the cues of a trustworthy collective unconscious that the individual already possesses. The mature individual or therapist is one who derives personal insight from dreams.

Much of contemporary personality theory assumes a human nature that is essentially trustworthy. In this case virtues are those traits that unfold as the self is actualized. It is assumed that the content of moral terms can be made specific by reference to abstract human nature, that there is consensus regarding the contour of this nature, and that it can be recognized by reference only to the individual self. The competent counselor, then, is one who is self-aware, and the self-aware therapist is one who will not unload his or her psychological baggage on unsuspecting clients.

Freedom

One last psychological assumption regarding the ideal character needs to be mentioned. I refer to the emphasis on freedom and autonomy as the focus of the moral life as particularly evident in existential psychologies. Morality is a consequence of personal choice. The character ideal is the individual whose life is truly free, who owns the responsibility of choice, and who rejects the imposition of values. Failure to grow personally is a function of our inability to take risks.

One does wonder at times whether the emphasis on the choice and freedom of healers is a consequence of a modern world in which individuals find themselves facing a plethora of options. In such a context it is not unreasonable to assume that the only thing one can be absolutely sure of is one's own autonomous choice. But choice in itself is empty and insufficient as a goal for character development. Freedom, in societies other than modern ones, has not necessarily been seen as an end in itself. Aristotle assumed that we become free as we develop the moral capability of guiding our own lives. Freedom lies not in making choices then, but rather in being the kind of person for whom some options are unacceptable. Hauerwas (1981) comments that we have made freedom the content of the moral life. The modern predicament is that while we are encouraged to make up our own minds, to choose our own morality, the price we pay is that the morality we choose does not obtain our full confidence.

Each of the above visions of healing character (analytic, self-aware, and free) limits the development of moral character. If character formation is simply a function of introspection, we divorce thought from practice. Clarification of values blatantly begs the question of which values are worth clarifying. The balance proposal fails to provide a defensible rationale for which forces are worth balancing. The individualism implicit in much psychological ideology works against the development of certain kinds of character because character is shaped by a larger, normative story and a communal praxis that is alien to these individualist assumptions. Lasch (1978) has remarked that the self, in a culture of narcissism, needs only to be clarified, not sacrificed to some ideal. I would submit that character is not so much a function of self-sufficiency or self-awareness, but of the kinds of *habits* we have acquired.

The Decline of the Enlightenment Project

One wonders on what bases ethical injunctions are made in the modern world. Sometimes ethical concerns are legitimated on the basis of the consequences of unethical behavior on the client or the therapist. At other times they are justified on the basis of professional role obligations and legal considerations. Occasionally there is some reference to contract as the basis of the therapeutic process. The clarification of an individual therapist's ethical principles and values is assumed critical.

In order to develop the model of the therapist as ethical agent, guardians of the profession have turned to the contribution of contemporary moral philosophy. Indeed, psychologists like Kohlberg (1968) have been relied on heavily as one model of moral inquiry. Kohlberg's model of how we engage in moral reasoning might serve as a systematic model for the development of therapists with ethical character. Though Kohlberg's model is familiar, I will review his stages of moral reasoning and apply the theory to therapists in terms of the development of character.

Kohlberg's theory describes the development of a general form of moral thought in terms of three major levels and six stages. I will describe each level and indicate the implications for the ethical development of psychotherapists.

1. *Preconventional Level.* At this level standards are perceived as external to the self. That which is morally right is demanded by power figures. Moral value resides in what good or bad acts are rewarded or punished. The process of moral reasoning at this level indicates a lack of awareness of the conventional rules of society. Conduct is modified by the influences of rewards and punishments. In stage one, physical consequences of action determine its goodness or badness. In stage two, right action is defined in terms of what instrumentally satisfied one's own needs. The therapist who functions at this level of morality engages in unethical behavior out of ignorance. Ethical commissions report that on occasion there are therapists who simply state that their behavior was not a violation of any regulation they were aware of. Or the therapist at this level reasons that, because there are negative consequences of an action (loss of license, litigation, imprisonment, loss of professional status, etc.), certain behaviors are wrong.

2. *Conventional Level:* At this level self is identified with social standards. The second level involves conformity to and maintenance of social standards and includes most adolescents and adults. Here conduct is controlled by the anticipation of social praise and blame. At this level, the expectations of family, group, or nation are the criteria of correct action. Specifically, stage three reasoning, usually referred to as the "good boy–nice girl" orientation, assumes that conformity to what is natural or stereotypical is good behavior. When applied to therapists, this mode of moral reasoning follows this pattern. What is right is right because most therapists do it. If most therapists accept gifts from clients, it is permissible. If most therapists are comfortable with developing friendships with former clients, then it is acceptable.

   A second stage (four) in this level of moral thought is more strongly identified with authority, fixed laws, and the maintenance of the social order. Therapists who function at this level are ethical because the law demands it. If suspicion of child abuse is to be reported, they report it because it is the law. If the laws of the land do not permit civil disobedience, these moral agents would expect clients to conform.

3. *Postconventional Level:* Self is differentiated from social standards in this level. Autonomous principles (e.g., justice) determine what is right at this level. A minority, however, while they accept the general *basic* moral principles that give rise to social rules, will choose on the basis of *personal* principles when conflict emerges between social and personal principles. In this third level, moral behavior is regulated by an ideal that transcends social praise and blame. Stage five reasoning posits that right action be defined as those general individual rights that have been critically examined and agreed upon by the whole society, e.g., the American Constitution.

The orientation of the last stage (six) defines that which is right in accord with self-chosen ethical principles that are comprehensive, consistent, and universal. These are not concrete rules (the Ten Commandments), but abstract principles (justice). If morality is adherence to abstract principles, then the ethical therapist is one who acts on principle with regard to such ethical issues as confidentiality, client autonomy and dependency, honesty about appropriate expectations regarding therapy, sexual relationships, reporting abuse, legitimate fees, licensure, deception, manipulation, accountability, etc.

Following Kohlberg, a therapist, at the highest level of moral development, would be one who acts autonomously on universalizable principles. For the therapist these rational principles might include the sanctity of life, the right to self-development, the right to fair treatment, etc. An alternative to this view assumes that character is constructed not only on the basis of abstract universal principles but on particular convictions that emerge out of the stories of particular communities.

Assumptions, Critique, and Alternatives

Transcendence and immanence, form and content, individual and community, reason and nature, freedom and necessity, universal and particular, unity and diversity, and ideal and real are dimensions not uncommon in ethical theory. Kohlberg casts his theory of moral development within these polarities, and that is already a commitment to a perspective that shapes his theory. Furthermore, his explicit bias is with the first term in each of the dimensions. Morality is grounded in the transcendence and obligation obtained from the universal structure of reason. The moral self finds its freedom and unity in the transcendent perspective and uniqueness of the individual personality.

But what then is the role of the opposite poles of the continua? By virtue of the fact that Kohlberg has constructed his theory by the first term, he has obviously granted their possibility, if not their existence. Are the two poles to be separated, integrated, held in tension, or ordered in priority? Kohlberg, at different times, does each of them. He wishes to maintain the integrity of the second terms since universal reason selects from diversity of moral content that which can be the basis of action. It is the free individual who transcends all communities and the necessity of nature. It is the moral self that gives unity to the diverse "selves": social, affective, and active.

The problem, however, is that Kohlberg's theory needs both terms. He needs transcendence to obtain obligation and a critique of the present state of nature. On the other hand, he needs the certainty and knowability that comes from that which is empirical, real. The former enables him to avoid irresponsibility and skepticism, individualism and relativism. However, without the latter his categories have no substance. The problem is then how Kohlberg can both hold separate *and* unite the two disparate poles. More specifically, the question is whether indeed Kohlberg's theory is grounded not on the transcendent, abstract ideals but on some particular content. Can he avoid the charge of provincialism? Does Kohlberg's moral self truly exhibit unity and not fragmentation?

Kohlberg's model of moral development is paradigmatically modern rather than premodern or postmodern. Implicitly, his Kantian model underlies most ethical discussions in the profession of psychotherapy. I will discuss the following assumptions that Kohlberg makes and the implications for professional character:

1. The focus of the ethical self is the rationality we have in common with all peoples.

2. The motivation of the moral self is not a critical variable.
3. The highest stage is moral autonomy. The individual is the locus of morality.
4. Moral inquiry as decisionism.

The Rational Self as Ethical

Kohlberg follows Kant in assuming that there is something in the nature of reason itself that operates on perception to create a sense of order. Knowledge is grounded in the structure of reason itself. Given the influence of Immanuel Kant, ethics is by nature universal rather than particular and it is assumed that individual ethical agents will know intuitively the meaning of ethical language (e.g., justice, fairness, etc.). Ethics is a matter of following moral principles that will reestablish harmony in the individual or society.

This universalist model has come under increasing criticism in the past decade by ethicists such as MacIntyre (1981), Stout (1988), and Hauerwas (1974, 1977, 1981, 1983). Stout (1988) refers to the kind of ethical language used in this model as moral Esperanto, an attempt to create a universal ethical language. Hauerwas (1983) challenges the universalist assumption: "All ethical reflection occurs relative to a particular time and place. Not only do ethical problems change from one time to the next but the very nature and structure of ethics is determined by the particularities of a community's history and convictions" (1983:1). MacIntyre (1981) indicates that in classical societies (Greco-Roman) morality is characterized by particularity and accountability. There is no desire to aspire to universality. From these societies, he suggests, we need to learn that "all morality is always to some degree tied to the socially local and particular and that the aspirations of the morality of modernity to a universality freed from all particularity is an illusion," and that "there is no way to possess the virtues except as part of a tradition in which we inherit them and our understanding of them from a series of predecessors in which heroic societies hold first place" (119).

The more extreme one is on the side of abstract reason the easier ethical formulas are to fill with *any* moral content. If reason provides no inherent basis for the choice of ends, the individual then tends to fill the vacuum with content derived either from personal experience or from common consensus of prevailing morality. Hence, MacIntyre has argued that

> The logical emptiness of the test of the categorical imperative is itself of social importance. Because the Kantian notion of duty is so formal that it can be given almost any content, it becomes available to provide sanction and a motive for the specific duties which any particular social and moral tradition may propose (1966:198).

It is a critical problem for Kohlberg if it can be shown that his theory is provincial rather than universal. Sullivan (1947) has pointed out correctly that Kohlberg identifies

> the process of 'universalization' with that of an 'impartial judge' in a jurisprudential procedure. This is possibly one of the reasons why stage 6 seems only present in Western cultural samples since stage 6 reflects a bias toward a jurisprudential process more prevalent in Western cultures. But can it be said that where that jurisprudential process is absent, that there is no attempt at universality? My own position is that Kohlberg and Rawls' process of universalization is sensitized to a juris-prudential model which is concretely developed in Western democracies and when this sensitivity is combined with other cultures lower on moral development, it is a culturally biased model (368).

Principles are abridgments of tradition (Stout, 1988). For those who know and accept the tradition the principles are useful. Browning (1976, 1988b) has repeatedly raised the question of the content of moral language and how that moral content is determined. The moral content of moral language is provided by a particular tradition. In the words of Jeffrey Stout (1988),

> Moral philosophy is not practiced from the vantage point of omniscience, above history. It begins, for any of us, at some particular site, where some moral languages are in use. . . . [Moral philosophy] is a kind of reflexive ethnography. It begins at home, with languages in use, and then reaches out to other possibilities, accessible from its particular historical position (72).

The Motivation of the Moral Self

What motivates and sustains movement through the stages of morality? Kohlberg's response to this question would be to point to the *natural* interaction of an active experiencing organism with its social environment that gives rise to the various types of moral reasoning. More specifically, development is a result of interaction between the universal internal features of the person's regulating tendencies and the universal features of the person's external social world. The growth of logical structures shapes the types of moral reasoning.

In Kohlberg's analysis and grounding of supreme moral categories emotions are irrelevant. Morality is not based on inclination or desire. Even if we were to grant that morality is not grounded on the emotive, it does not follow that the path from the moral ideal to action might not include passion. Thus, while Kant wanted unity and spontaneity, the result was more aptly described as fragmentation and, subsequently, self-conscious morality. Kohlberg's theory of moral development seems to reflect these tensions in Kant. An intrinsic connection between reason and will is assumed in the mature moral individual. Kohlberg admits that there are those who know what should be done according to the moral principle, but don't do it. Nonetheless, he would maintain that true knowledge of principles of justice predicts virtuous action. In this model emotion is an irrational process and Kohlberg finds no significant role for emotional identification in the development of morality.

Autonomy and Relatedness

Kohlberg's moral self is transcendent not only because reason is universal but also because it transcends all communities. The stage six person operates from a position that is prior to all communal claims to authority. The moral individual is then autonomous and free.

There has been a major challenge to an ethic of character that assumes that autonomy is the focal point of moral agency. In her research, Carol Gilligan (1981) used the moral dilemmas developed by Lawrence Kohlberg with women instead of men. She found that in women's analysis of moral situations there was an emphasis on conflicting responsibilities in the context of caring relationships. Using Kohlberg's (1968) data as the basis, she observed that men focused on fairness in the context of competing rights. Women embedded their discussion of morality in a narrative context while men embedded it in an abstract and formal context. Women seemed to assume that the world coheres because there is a matrix of relationships rather than a system of rules. Men assumed that conflict can be resolved by logical deduction. Law mediates the dispute. Moral conflict is an impersonal conflict of claims, abstracted from history and a network of relationships.

Decisionism

Contemporary moral philosophy tends to assume that one's moral theory emerges in terms of a rational response to specific moral problems. Ethics then is concerned primarily with ambiguous situations or hard decisions. The emphasis on moral quandaries fails to examine the ethical in terms of a larger perspective of lifestyle. The ethical agent is one who solves moral problems. The religious healer or therapist is then one who deals largely with ethical problems requiring decisions: abortion, divorce, career choice, individuation from one's family, religious values. Decisionism focuses on how to resolve ethical decisions, not on who the persons are who make the decisions. Decisionism is parasitic. It depends on previous moral education that already produces moral characters capable of moral decisions.

In this chapter I have attempted to critically examine the effect of Kohlberg's commitment to formalist ethics on his formulation of the nature of morality and its implications for therapy. Though Kohlberg's categories of universal, principled, morality, and autonomy have some similarity to the Judeo-Christian concepts of transcendence and immanence, and of wholeness and freedom, they are not identical. It is when Kohlberg fills his categories with specific content that tension emerges in his own theoretical system and that the contrast with Christianity is greatly increased.

In the next chapter I attempt to outline an alternative model of the self that is more communal and relational. It is an effort to build on the first two sections of the book that assume an ethical culture and community as the context of the individual therapist.

10

Pastoring Our
Personal Congregations

The language of the soul has gone the way of Edsels and hula-hoops. Barrett (1986) suggests we no longer have a language of the soul in psychology. It may be that existentially the souls of those who are therapists and Christians are alive and well. However, one would hardly know it from a perusal of the writings of Christians in psychology, from the continuing reports of sexual violations by religious psychotherapists, and from the paucity of reflections by Christian psychologists on the subject of the soul. The transformation of our souls depends on our openness to the God who is transforming and requires a lexicon of the self that enables us to recognize the nature of that transformation. Perhaps, then, we as therapists will be more open to the work of the Holy Spirit in learning and healing. Care of the soul, I believe, will result in character.

If there is a loss of soul or a loss of a language of the soul, I would expect that imagination would be a scarce commodity, that artistry would not be encouraged. Psychotherapy is as much an art as it is a science. Indeed, an artistic perspective of the self struggles for recognition and support in the larger psychological community. Psychotherapy requires moral imagination. A religion of obedience does not necessarily foster creativity and imagination.

Loss of soul and loss of a language of the soul are not independent. The increasing lapses among psychologists in sexual ethics points to the emptiness of the soul. The story that I hear from those who have engaged in sexually inappropriate behavior is that they knew there was this other part of them that acted in clearly inappropriate ways, but they seemed helpless to do anything about it. They felt very needy but had no way of expressing the need and assumed that another person could sexually fill the void.

In this chapter I wish to extend the notions of culture, community, and character to a model of the self. The "self" that emerges from this perspective is to be one capable of ethical discernment and religious character (Sanford, 1970). As indicated in earlier chapters, I am less than satisfied with any model of the self that is not communal (O'Connor, 1981). Therapists need a vocabulary and grammar of the soul that incorporates individual and communal dimensions. I want to argue that our sense of self is constitutionally social. The individual is composed of a myriad of internal subpersonalities. In this model we are all perambulating congregations.

A corollary of this first proposition of the communal self is that the relationship between internal selves is destructive when the ethic that shapes their relationships is unjust. The ethic that governs the external Christian community is just as *apropos* to the internal selves as it is to historical communities. I wish to argue that the ethic of the Reign of God is an ethic that is applicable to the healthy internal as well as the historically real congregation. A further implication is that personal growth involves the integration of the conflicting introjected personalities that result from developmental process and from life in a pluralistic society. What could be more consistent with the goals of therapy and the Reign of God than to resolve conflict by dialogue, to make our enemies our friends, not only externally but internally as well? Ultimately, to say that God is One should suggest that psychological unity is better than fragmentation. To say that God is manifest as Three—Father, Son, and Holy Spirit—is an affirmation of diversity within unity.

Communal Self

It should come as no surprise that just as the West assumes the individual is the center point of society, it also assumes that the individual is indivisible. The Enlightenment assumed that the ego was unitary. In his *An Essay on Human Understanding,* John Locke (1690/1964) included a chapter (27) entitled "On Identity and Diversity." He began by asserting that the human sense of identity emerges from our ability to compare things over time. Of God, he stated that "God is without beginning, eternal, unalterable, and everywhere, and therefore concerning his identity there can be no doubt" (207). Of matter, vegetables, and animals, Locke stated that they too remain the same. Then he draws the implications for personhood.

> This also shows wherein the identity of the same man consists: viz., in nothing but a participation of the same continued life, by constantly fleeting particles of matter, in succession vitally united to the same organized body. He that shall place the identity of man in anything else, but like that of other animals, in one fitly organized body, taken in any one instant, and from thence continued, under one organization of life, in several successively fleeting particles of matter united to it, will find hard to make an embryo, one of years, mad or sober, the same man (210).

He defined the person as a "thinking intelligent being, that has reason and reflection, and can consider itself as itself, the same thinking thing, in different times and places; which it does only by that consciousness which is inseparable from thinking, and, as it seems to me, essential to it; it being impossible for anyone to perceive without perceiving that he does perceive" (211). The drunk and the sober individual are the same person. The consciousness of each is identical.

It is the precisely opposite perspective that I wish to explore. Various psychologists implicitly or explicitly have played with the notion of the plural self. From James and Freud onward the assumption of one coherent self has been questioned. Whether it was the presence of the unconscious or the movement between stages of development, the self was not assumed to be as integrated as was commonly believed. Systemic family therapists/theorists have recently pointed to the family within that may well mirror the external family (Schwartz, 1987, 1988a, 1988b, 1988c; Bryant, Kessler, and Shirar, 1992). Object relations theorists would understand (Greenberg and Mitchell, 1983; Cashdan, 1988); we are all products of significant introjects. Symbolic interactionists would also share this perspective (Mead, 1934). Who we become grows out of our interactions with others and those interactions are supported by language. Jungian narratives are helpful (Bly, 1990; Estes, 1992). My many selves are then personified archetypes. Jung called them the "little people." Inner struggles are a conflict between different personalities. The more narrow stories of the behaviorist are of some help. Different situations and persons reinforce and evoke different response patterns. Even biologically oriented psychologists like Gazzaniga (1985) and Ornstein (1986) argue that there are independent centers in the brain that permit independent characters to emerge.

Sociological analyses of postmodernity also support a multiple perspective on the self. It is possible that our souls mirror the larger pluralist society. What I do in everyday life is reflected in my soul. But it is not just the problem of living in a pluralist world that creates pluralist selves. It is also a matter of what kind of selves this world creates and we introject. If in everyday life I am a part of an oppressive male culture, in my soul I will tend to dismiss the feminine as well. If I am a part of a social hierarchy that declares who is important and who is not, I am confident that there is a similar hierarchy in my inner world of personalities.

One person who has been most articulate in developing a communal and ethical model of the self has been the Russian writer Georges Gurdjieff (Ouspensky, 1949). His fundamental assumption was that "To speak the truth one must know what the truth is and what a lie is, and first of all in oneself" (22). One of the lies he felt we lived with was the deception of the unitary "I." The self is a plurality. We are never the same for long. We are continually changing. The following quote sparkles with possibilities:

> We think that if a man is called Ivan he is always Ivan. Nothing of the kind. Now he is Ivan, in another minute he is Peter, and a minute later he is Nicholas, Sergius, Matthew, Simon. And all of you think he is Ivan. You know that Ivan cannot do a certain thing. He cannot tell a lie for instance. Then you find he has told a lie and you are surprised he could have done so. And, indeed, Ivan cannot lie and you are surprised he could have done so. And, indeed, Ivan cannot lie; it is Nicholas who lied. And when the opportunity presents itself Nicholas cannot *help lying*. You

will be astonished when you realize what a multitude of these Ivans and Nicholasses live in one man. If you learn to observe them there is no need to go to a cinema (1949:53, emphasis his).

Each of the personalities calls itself "I," each assumes to be the master, and none will recognize the other. When each gets to be king for a day (or less), they pass edicts and conduct business as they please without regard to the others. The others have to pay for the mistakes made, sometimes for the rest of their lives. Each part thinks it is the whole.

A Communal Ethic for a Communal Self

How do the multiple selves get along? Is there community? Is there unity or is there conflict? Is there coherence or fragmentation? Is there justice or injustice? Is there narcissism or a commitment to service among the selves? Permit me an illustration. Imagine a male psychologist and therapist (I know males better) teaching at a graduate institution of psychology, whose self has various parts, dimensions, or personalities. I will call him Michael. He prepares diligently for his lectures, presents enthusiastically, and his students admire him. This is Michael's most public and most developed self. Spiritually this personality gets excited about God the creator. His tragic flaw is the arrogance that comes with the power of knowledge. Then there is Michael the cook, the baker of foods—by recipe of course. Spiritually this Michael thinks there is a very practical side to Christianity. Somehow, being a Christian should make a difference in how we live. The tragic flaw of this self is that he oversimplifies what may be more complex. There is the Michael who appears only when he is with his parents. He is more docile, less talkative. It is almost as if his personality stopped growing after he left home twenty years ago. Michael is a licensed psychologist and has a small private practice. As therapist he tends to gravitate toward cognitive-behavioral approaches to change. He observes that some of his clients change, but wonders why he is not more spontaneous, imaginative, and creative in his therapy.

There is another personality that Michael will not even recognize as legitimate. She comes to him in dreams. Her beauty and sexuality frighten him. She is inspiring, poetic, and gracious. This is a very fragile self, easily run over by other personalities. If Michael were to listen to her, his spirituality and therapy would be different. He might be less analytical, more open to diversity, and more relaxed. Then there is his neglected self that often acts like a hurt child. This one is still angry at his pious but distant Christian parents. This self can be cruel, filled with hate. Michael's other personalities are more fragmentary. There are some sudden mood swings, occasional posturing, some clowning, and the ethnic self that appears only on Saturday night.

There is one more personality: the executive. This is the personality the person with a multiple personality disorder truly lacks and desperately seeks. At best this personality creates order, pastors the congregation of selves. At worst the executive is the one who exiles some personalities, destroys others, toadies to one and humors another. It is what I would call the Constantinian personality. It rules by force; it rejects diversity. The notion that there is a single autonomous "I" that organizes our life and activities is a dangerous myth. This monolithic self tends to assume more organization than is really there. It reflects the arrogance of the modern world. That is another version of individualism. It is the executive personality in Michael that is most easily seduced into thinking we are able to create order and to do so alone. Michael's self needs to be pastored by being reminded that only God is one.

Each of our personalities by virtue of its character can create conflict. It does so through its style of communication, idiosyncrasies, temperament, abilities, functions, autonomy, attitudes, and worldview. One can be dogmatic, the other tolerant. One patient, another very impatient. One is saintly, another is pagan. One part panders to other's wishes, another says no. One is arrogant, another is hypercritical of the self. One part celebrates, another holds a pity party. One can be legalistic, the other all grace. Some of these may not be full-blown personalities. Some are just voices, fragments of memories, sudden impulses, images that flit through my mind and shape my behavior.

In this model the difference between health and its opposite is that in the case of the latter the various selves may be so terrifying or out of control that working and maintaining relationships is impossible. Those who are deeply troubled know they cannot hold it all together.

Gurdjieff speaks of the many conflicting selves within in terms of a distinction between various levels of consciousness within the self. At the lowest level there is a passive state—sleep. Physically we spend a third of our life there and, he suggests, most of our waking life as well, unless we wake up. A second level is referred to as 'clear consciousness.' It is in this state in which people

> walk the streets, write books, talk on lofty subjects, take part in politics, kill one another, [and] which they regard as active and call 'clear consciousness' or the 'waking state of consciousness.' The term 'clear consciousness' or 'waking state of consciousness' seems to have been given in jest, especially when you realize what *clear consciousness* ought in reality to be and what the state in which man lives and acts really is (Ouspensky 1949:141, emphasis his).

Gurdjieff comments on the war raging at the time he was teaching (WWI) as follows: "Let us take some event in the life of humanity. For instance, war. There is a war going on at the present moment. What does it signify? It signifies that several millions of sleeping people are trying to destroy several millions of other sleeping people. They would not do this, of course, it they were to wake up" (143). Gurdjieff encouraged his disciples to remember themselves, to be conscious of themselves. To remember oneself is to remember oneself as one is observing oneself. The opposite is to live and act and reason in deep sleep. To remember ourselves takes conscious effort so we can awake. Gurdjieff makes the point that we make constant identifications with the external world, and these objections of identification change. "A man identifies with a small problem which confronts him and he completely forgets the great aims with which he began his work. He identifies with one thought and forgets other thoughts; he has identified with one feeling, with one mood, and forgets his own wider thoughts, emotions and moods" (Ouspensky, 1949:150).

For me, a major source of understanding for the conflicted plural self comes from my clients. There have been those who suffered with multiple personality disorder. Briefly stated, the emergence of several distinct personalities comes as a result of traumatic events. These individuals found their sense of self shattered. The trauma experienced could come from being a victim of serious physical and sexual abuse, or being a witness to the atrocities of the Khmer Rouge regime. In order to survive once the central self is destroyed, other personalities emerge to take its place. Each personality has its own way of thinking, feeling, and acting. Each may even have its own physiology: blood pressure, heart rate, food preferences, and sleep patterns. Some are protectors, others are persecutors, one compulsive, the other chaotic, some male, some female. Sometimes one takes over control, sometimes another. Developing a core sense of self is a long excruciating pilgrimage.

In the 1950s a person with many personalities was considered a rarity, and so we too-quickly considered them either psychotic or demon possessed. When we begin creating categories of us and them (we are normal and they are not), I become suspicious. Paul reminds us in his letter to the Corinthians that there is a commonality to the weaknesses we ALL experience (1 Cor. 10:13). In a sense we all have fragmented personalities within us. We are all constitutionally social.

There can be little question that the ancient Hebrew soul is both a unified self and a conflicted one. On the one hand, Hebrews did not make the metaphysical distinction between mind and body so common in the Hellenistic literature (Wolff, 1974; Whitlock, 1960). Yet in the creation account we have the following:

> Then God said, "Let us make man in our image, in our likeness, and let them rule over the fish of the sea and the birds of the air, over the livestock, over all the earth, and over all the creatures that move along the ground." So God created man in his own image, in the image of God he created him; male and female he created them (Gen. 1:26–27).

One way of reading this text is that the image of God in humanity is relational. God says, "Let *us* make humanity in *our* likeness." One could argue that the plurality in the Godhead is reflected in a relationality in humanity. I wish to go a step further and argue that at one level the multiple self is also a reflection (image) of the triune God.

There is also a fundamental tension in the Hebrew soul. That tension is between good and evil, between what we are called to be and what we realize we are. I am reminded of the apostle Paul's own comments on his conflicted multiple self: "So I find this law at work: When I want to do good, evil is right there with me. For in my inner being I delight in God's law; but I see another law at work in the members of my body, waging war against the law of my mind and making me a prisoner of the law of sin at work within my members" (Rom. 7:21–23).

Then there is the parable Jesus told his disciples about the wheat and tares that seems relevant.

> Jesus told them another parable: "The kingdom of heaven is like a man who sowed good seed in his field. But while everyone was sleeping, his enemy came and sowed weeds among the wheat, and went away. When the wheat sprouted and formed heads, then the weeds also appeared. The owner's servants came to him and said, 'Sir, didn't you sow good seed in your field? Where then did the weeds come from?' 'An enemy did this,' he replied. The servants asked him, 'Do you want us to go and pull them up?' 'No,' he answered, 'because while you are pulling the weeds, you may root up the wheat with them. Let both grow together until the harvest. At that time I will tell the harvesters: First collect the weeds and tie them in bundles to be burned; then gather the wheat and bring it into my barn'" (Matt. 13:24–30).

What an interesting parable. It is not clear what exactly Jesus meant by the wheat and the weeds, but it is clear one was acceptable (grain) and one was not (weeds). Perhaps our personalities are like good grain and weeds that grow up together. Indeed, in other contexts, Jews made a distinction between *yetzer ara* and *yetzer tov,* good and evil within the soul. I am reminded of the argument in the book of James (4:1) for why war emerges: "What causes fights and quarrels among you? Don't they come from your desires that battle within you?"

I would like to argue that all that I have said in the earlier sections about the nature of the Reign of God and the calling of the church applies to the congregation within. Just as there is a need for a corporate ethic there is a need for a communal ethic for ourselves. All that writers in the Believer's Church tradition have said about the ethic that is to govern the life of the church community (Gish, 1979; Hauerwas, 1981) can be applied to the internal community. What Paul writes about in terms of the church applies to the internal congregation.

> For by the grace given me I say to every one of you: Do not think of yourself more highly than you ought, but rather think of yourself with sober judgment, in accordance with the measure of faith God has given you. Just as each of us has one body with many members, and these members do not all have the same function, so in Christ we who are many form one body, and each member belongs to all the others. We have different gifts, according to the grace given us. If a man's gift is prophesying, let him use it in proportion to his faith. If it is serving, let him serve; if it is teaching, let him teach; if it is encouraging, let him encourage; if it is contributing to the needs of others, let him give generously; if it is leadership, let him govern diligently; if it is showing mercy, let him do it cheerfully. Love must be sincere. Hate what is evil; cling to what is good. Be devoted to one another in brotherly love. Honor one another above yourselves. . . . Live in harmony with one another. Do not be proud, but be willing to associate with people of low position. Do not be conceited (Rom. 12:3–10, 16).

One part of the tension between our many selves is a product of history: one self values thinking and another feeling. Another part of the tension of the selves is ethical: one self violates another. When we apply a New Testament ethic to the internal selves, this would suggest that the arrogance of the executive be avoided, that some selves should be honored, that the diversity is good. In sum, the ethic of the Reign of God that governs the church governs the self.

The present world is incredibly fragmenting and traumatizing. Increasingly we are told that we live in a world that is pluralistic. In a given day we travel through a myriad of different communities, each with their own demands, expectations, and loyalties. How many times have we not been told that we live in a fragmented world? Well, if we live in a fragmented world why do we assume that we are integrated and immune to its fragmenting forces? One of our tasks as therapists is to tend to our souls, to pastor our inner congregations so character and unity can emerge.

In the first part of this chapter I was concerned only to make the point that the self is multiple and that unity is an illusion. In this second part I have asserted that there is a diversity that may well reflect the Godhead, and at the same time this diversity may be a fundamental conflict among the selves, a conflict that can be assessed ethically. In the following section I wish to suggest an approach to change that is ethically and communally motivated. As therapists, and simply as human beings, we are called to personal unity and to enjoy diversity.

The Unified Self and the God Who Is One

Therapists too need the healing touch of God. We will need to pastor all of these personalities in order for the image of God to be more evident in our lives. Inner unity will come as we wrestle with the suffering of that which pulls us to "yes" and "no" within. Gurdjieff suggested that there are at least four selves: a carnal self (the body), a natural self (feelings, desires), a spiritual self (mind), and a divine spiritual self (unified I). The latter self is able to work on the previous three simultaneously. To obtain this fourth way one must be very serious about embracing all sides of oneself. One must live in conditions that do not render it impossible. This fourth way has no definite forms like the others. Working on the fourth way affects all the other ways as well.

Gurdjieff points out that achieving the spiritual psyche requires fusion by means of hard inner work and struggle. Inner unity is obtained by friction, by struggle between "yes" and "no" in the person. It takes sacrifice and the rejection of comfort to attain unity. Immortality on earth is a kind of individuality and inner unity; it is a permanent and unchangeable "I," consciousness, and will. Real "I" can emerge only from one's essence. Gurdjieff makes a distinction between essence and personality. Essence is what is one's own. Personality is what is not one's own. Personality comes from outside, from what one has learned. In most cases the personality is the active element in the person while the essence is the passive element. Personality is a result of the roles or buffers that result from the work of the various selves.

The essence of the moral self (Kohlberg's language), or the soul, I see in terms of the *imago dei,* the image of God in the self. This is real Self (Barth, 1961). As a result, the executive personality needs to hear that only God is one. Some personalities like Christ, need to be given a body, to be incarnated so they can be seen and understood. Other need the energy of the Holy Spirit. It seems all of our personalities need to hear the good news of our Triune God.

In the parable noted above (Matt. 13:24–30), the servants want impulsively to tear out the weeds together with the grain, much like a sectarian psychologist might. But the wise owner realizes that to pull up the weeds means some grain will also be lost. Perhaps it is like that with our souls as well. We will need to live patiently with those selves we think are weeds. To converse with those parts will then mean patience, not passivity. It is not always clear which personalities are grain and which are weeds. Sometimes a weed turns out to be a gift. Listening to the pained self may reveal a reason why it is pained. There will come a time when the good and not so good will be separated. Then that which is truly evil will be destroyed. But not yet. We must live with the tension and learn to live in peace. Jesus reminds us not to "resist one who is evil" (Matt. 5:39).

The centered heart is one that moves toward greater unity. Just as Jesus prays for the unity of the church, we must pray for the unity of our souls. After all, Paul reminds us: "There is one body and one Spirit—just as you were called to one hope when you were called—one Lord, one faith, one baptism; one God and Father of all, who is over all and through all and in all" (Eph. 4:4–6). While we live in this clay vessel we will always be fragmented, it is a gift and a problem. I am created with the potential of being a multiple self with all its rich diversity, but I am called to be whole, one just as God is one (Mark 12:29; Rom. 3:30; 1 Cor. 8:6; 1 Tim. 2:5; James 2:19). So when we struggle toward wholeness, the image of God becomes clearer in our lives. Only God is one. Oneness and centeredness is a gift and what we strive for, not something we assume in advance. The heart that is focused is more unified. To quote Kierkegaard, "Purity of heart is to will one thing." The heart that is pastored has a deeper peace.

A communal psychology would then be one that invites us to pastor, to listen, and to dialogue with all of our many selves so that unity and diversity are respected. An ethic that governs the life of the external and internal congregation might require the following:

1. To encourage respect for one another.
2. To treat each member equally.
3. To confront persons who dominate and overrule.
4. To facilitate reconciliation where there is conflict.
5. To empower the weak, give them voice.
6. To confront evil rather than denying it.
7. To call a meeting when necessary.

I posit that by analogy the ethic that governs the church is also appropriate to the internal congregation.

To Encourage Respect for One Another

Just as Jew and Gentile have a legitimate place beside each other, so also our various personalities need to be recognized. It will mean that I recognize and give names to the personalities that are creative and those that are destructive. If to pastor means to encourage respect for one another in our churches, the same applies to our inner congregation. Too often we simply dismiss persons as possessors of strange ideas or quirky dispositions. When we pastor ourselves we must assume that all the personalities have a right to be recognized, though not necessarily to be condoned (both wheat and weeds). My angry self is not my total self nor is my altruistic self. Is it possible that we are in fact so created as to be able to have more than one personality and that it is not automatically a sign of our fallenness or of pathology? Diversity can be a gift in a church and in an inner congregation. The problem may not lie in the diversity but in the inability to pastor them so as to create unity. As therapists, to show respect for our multiple selves means that a mood deserves to be made into a personality so that a conversation can go on. We will understand ourselves better if we make concrete our fragmented personality.

To Treat Each Member Equally

The writer of the book of James (James 2) warns not to give preference to the rich. By analogy we would then not give preference to some selves and reject others. If, in our churches, to pastor means we will not prefer one member to another, either to victimize or to venerate, then we will not simply scapegoat or idolize one of the personalities. Just as we scapegoat individuals in communities and families, therapists can blame one part of themselves for all of their therapeutic failures. Just as we can glorify one member in the congregation, we can excessively admire one of our successful therapeutic personalities. We tend to mistake our parts for the whole, a kind of psychological synecdoche.

To Confront Persons Who Dominate and Overrule

We are called to confront persons who dominate and overrule in the church; so also in our personal congregation. In therapy one self needs to be asked to speak less, perhaps to be silent for a while. For some therapists it may be the intellectual personality that needs attention, for others the pragmatic one, and yet others the too sensitive relational one.

To Facilitate Reconciliation Where There Is Conflict

Matthew 18 suggests that when there is conflict we are invited to facilitate reconciliation between persons. Our inner congregation often needs reconciliation. Just as there are coalitions among family members to overpower another member, so also there are coalitions among our subselves. Such coalitions escalate the conflict and the issue needs to be addressed. That sexual self that seems uncontrollable needs to be pastored, talked to, cared for, not exiled, ostracized, or excommunicated. After all, Paul sought to reconcile Jew and Gentile.

To Empower the Weak, To Give Them Voice

Without question, to pastor means to empower the weak, to give them voice. For some, that rejected personality is the more quiet, poetic, and artistic one, while for others, the repudiated self is one who is a thinker, public, and assertive. If one wonders where the rejected personality is, one needs to ask what criticism hurts most. What can get me most angry? If we follow the trail we may find a frightened child, a dependent adolescent, or perhaps a fearful parent.

The self we go public with is the one that is often most developed. However, Paul points out in talking of Jesus that the stone that the builders rejected became the cornerstone of the church. The race is not necessarily won by the swift. The Old Testament reminds us to be hospitable to strangers, they could be angels. Perhaps that applies to members in our personal inner congregation as well. That part of me that I consider the weakest may in fact be the one through whom God will meet me, through whom may come spiritual renewal. Then the last shall be first.

To Confront Evil Rather Than Denying It

Just as in the church we must confront evil rather than denying it, so also in our personal congregation. When there is sexual impropriety in the Corinthian church, Paul calls on the church to address the problem. There are parts of our selves we all fear to face. They are the enemy. We prefer problems be out of sight and out of mind. That has been applied to people we don't like and can be applied to the inner people we don't like. Am I willing to admit that there is even a barbaric member in my personal congregation, one who can be cruel, one who can abuse? Is it possible that in our dreams some character perpetrates acts of unmitigated evil. If so, I assume that personality is part of my psyche. If we are to love and pray for our enemies, I think it is appropriate to do so within as well.

To Call a Meeting When Necessary

In the early church when there was a problem, a meeting was called (Acts 15). We, too, can call a meeting, an inner meeting of the members. I realize a boring church business meeting is not exactly a good analogy for the meeting of inner selves. However, we will not learn how to get along with each other unless all members are present and they communicate with each other. So to pastor our inner congregation may also mean calling a meeting, an inner meeting of the members. Sometimes it is useful to write out a script in which every member's comments are recorded on paper (Johnson, 1986). For others it means quiet meditation.

I began this chapter concerned that we need a more differentiated language of the soul, one that enables us to talk more articulately of our pain, one that facilitates change, one that is sensitive to artistic metaphors and encourages creativity, one that is ethically and communally sensitive, one that does not absolutize volition, and one that is gender sensitive. To think I have fulfilled this task would be to pander to the hubris of my executive personality. I hope to have made a beginning.

Some cautions. The use of the metaphor of the communal self must not be reified. It is intended as a useful fiction. If it is not helpful in becoming more deeply Christian in character, then we need a different psychology. But we need one. Furthermore, with Gurdjieff, I believe that a person cannot waken by him or herself. One person awakes and wakens the others. Christ's disciples even slept when he was praying in the Garden of Gethsemene for the last time. Given the complexity of the self, it is impossible for us to know ourselves by ourselves. That is the role of the teacher and the friend. The reason is that we do not remember ourselves. We need the community of God's people to help us be aware of our many selves and hold us accountable to an ethic that brings personal and cultural peace. The church can be a school in which people are trained to live with their many selves.

If as therapists we value only our intellectual personality, in all probability we will neglect the sensitive, feeling side that needs an embodiment, acceptance, and nurture. And if it is not nurtured, that feeling side has a way of distorting even our best ideas. If in therapy I live out my feeling personality only, to respond confidently to the intellectual client may create considerable anxiety. If I don't take care of the weakest member I tend to project it onto others.

To work at pastoring my personal congregation might be another meaning for Paul's encouragement to work out our salvation with fear and trembling—i.e., seriously. In the Believers' Church tradition there is an emphasis on community, and that service and discipleship can lead to healthy communal life. I could not agree more. What we need, however, is a communal view of the self. The Believers' Church tradition has a most limited vocabulary for the self. And furthermore, the very ethic I have learned from my Believers' Church heritage of peace, voluntarism, and discipleship is appropriate for how I treat each of my many selves.

Conclusion: Experiences between Jerusalem and Athens

This book grew out of both experience and reflection. Let me conclude with the experiences from which the reflections emerged. How has my character been shaped by the cultures and communities that I have been a part of? How has the contour of my character been influenced? How are the yearnings of my heart a reflection of the Reign of God? Can I as a professional open my experiences and praxis to the discernment of a group of believers?

This chapter will detail my many expeditions between Athens and Jerusalem. The structure of the chapter follows the structure of this book. It tells of my movement away from a provincial identity. Perhaps in my journey I have developed a more global perspective. Slowly I have come to recognize and appreciate my own ethnoreligious story. I hope the experience of membership in the church and specific Christian communities has tempered my ego. The meaning of being both a professional psychologist and a Christian has become clearer. This chapter recounts my struggle to allow a different kind of masculinity to emerge. Clients and dreams have had a transforming impact. Other Christian traditions have made me more aware of the importance of symbols and beauty. I trust that the account of my pilgrimage communicates the joy and struggle of relating ethics to culture, community, and character.

Culture: An International Identity

While teaching at Tabor College, and again at Fresno Pacific College, I took groups of students to Guadalajara and Mexico City. Both were life-changing experiences as we struggled to learn the language and the culture. The Orozco and Rivera paintings integrated art and politics. The evangelical missionaries taking language study with us were so dogmatic and ethnocentric, that I was embarrassed for the witness of the church (Dueck, 1983, 1985).

In the fall of 1989 I was given one of those once-in-a-lifetime opportunities: to travel to the then Soviet Union. Mennonite Health Services organized an exchange program and a group of twenty mental health professionals toured the country. We observed firsthand the Soviet mental health programs. The Soviet Union has played a significant role in my life. My parents were born in the Ukraine. My grandmother told me stories about life in the "old country." My mother-in-law wrote letters faithfully to relatives in the USSR from the 1930s to the 1990s, when she was finally able to visit them in Germany. I could understand U.S. antipathy for Soviet authoritarianism but I could never endorse U.S. militarism (Dueck, 1983). These people too are made in the image of God. So for me to step on Russian soil was another kind of homecoming.

The first week was spent traveling in the Ukraine. I saw the village my forbears had built. But there were no Mennonites left. After the second world war Stalin had resettled all German-speaking Ukrainians to the interior. A local museum carried a few pieces of Mennonite culture. A hundred years of labor reduced to a dinner plate and some clothing! As I traveled through the villages I remembered how as a four-year-old my wife's father saw his own father shot in front of him.

It was the Baptist conference that arranged our visit to the mental health agencies in Moscow. The pastor was eager to show off Western mental health professionals who were Christians. The most interesting of experiences was the Kaschenko hospital where the women from the Baptist congregation had been volunteering for the past two years. The Kaschenko hospital in Moscow is one of the oldest (1894) and largest (2600 beds) psychiatric hospitals in the Soviet Union. The catchment area for the hospital was approximately two million people. Patients were placed in wards according to the specific area from which they came. I was told there were patients who indicated that they wished to get into the wards where the Baptist volunteers were working.

Dr. Kozyrev, the clinical director, placed much emphasis on the importance of social rehabilitation of patients. He was concerned that psychiatry had lost its emphasis on the importance of prevention. He also indicated that the most pressing problems for him were financing the hospital, developing new ideas, and the slow pace at which psychiatry was changing. He indicated that, before they had political problems; now they have economic problems. With the dissolution of the USSR and its current economic problems I can only imagine their distress today.

The evidences of *perestroika* were evident at the hospital. First, the openness of our own meeting was evidence. Second, there was a less formal atmosphere at the hospital. Third, wards could decide on a treatment program and initiate new ideas. One ward was organized according to a collective, but patients were promised that the products of their labor (clothing for children) would be sold and that the profits would be returned to individual patients. Also, the old concrete walls outside were being removed and wrought iron fences were replacing them. One also sensed that administration was more open to ideas that came up from the various staff.

The question was raised regarding involuntary hospitalization of political dissidents. Kozyrev and his assistant were visibly pained by the question. They indicated that part of the problem was that the press had distorted the situation at least in part. They did admit that in times past there had been involuntary hospitalizations for political reasons. They hoped that we would not judge the services of the hospital on the basis of past history. The day we left, the World Health Organization reinstated the Soviet representatives as full members. Everyone rejoiced. But the question of the relation of ethics to therapy and culture remained.

One of the highlights of our stay at this hospital was the meeting with several hundred staff members. Kozyrev opened the meeting with a moment of silence for victims of the earthquake in California that had occurred the day before. Kozyrev read translated summaries of our vitae and then opened the meeting for questions. The audience was lively. Questions revolved around ethical issues in America, treatment approaches, and so forth. After the meeting, Pastor Zhidkov, the organizer from the Baptist conference, indicated that the meeting was without question historic. This was the first time in the history of the hospital that staff had been invited to a consultation such as this. Also, most of those staff present had probably never before met educated believers who were also professional mental health practitioners. It was quite clear that Zhidkov was proud to show off his American friends who were both Christians and professional psychologists.

Culture: Crossing the Color Barrier

My convictions have changed over the years, largely because of experiences and relationships that have forced reassessment. A most significant event occurred the summer before entering graduate school. I had been accepted into the graduate psychology program at the University of Manitoba and would be conducting research in learning with the proverbial white rat as subject. But Anne and I received an invitation to assist a group of African-American Mennonite churches in North Carolina. The conference numbered 200 members in seven small churches and were spread across 200 square miles. We accepted.

It was all new: our first extended trip into the United States; the first time we crossed the Mason-Dixon line into the American south; the first thirty-six hour bus ride anywhere; the first encounter with red clay that would not wash out; our first experience with African-American Mennonites. What happened was entirely unexpected. We helped out with camp work and at the end of the summer the church leaders invited us to return. That an African-American community would invite us to live with them was overwhelming. We were honored. I quickly applied to the counseling program at Appalachian State University in Boone and was accepted with a teaching assistantship position as a bonus. The church leadership asked us to work with the young people and assist in pastoring the churches. We were excited.

April, 1968. The wooden casket carrying Martin Luther King moved slowly across the screen of our little black and white TV. Reverend Rhondo Horton, the conference leader, and his wife, "Miz" Ruth, were with us. There couldn't have been a starker contrast. They were dark skinned, we were white. They had sharecropped with their parents at the turn of the century. We grew up in the 1950s in Mennonite homes. For years Reverend Rhondo had hauled coal from the Virginia mines. We had attended college. They knew unconsciously where the color boundary was in every public place, whether restroom or restaurant. We barely knew where the Mason-Dixon line was. "Miz" Ruth sat there dabbing at her eyes with her white handkerchief. Reverend Rhondo cried openly. We sat quietly. For both of them Martin Luther King had been a modern Moses.

In Boone, North Carolina, where we lived those two years, the African-American neighborhood was small and conspicuous in a predominantly white county. When we arrived in the late 1960s the young people in our church had never bowled in the local bowling alley. They had eaten in the local restaurant only a year earlier. They had never seen a movie in the local theater. Such blatant prejudice was simply not part of our repertoire of experience. Or perhaps I had been blind to it in Winnipeg, Manitoba, Canada. There was the time we went swimming at an all white beach. When we arrived some thirty strong, the beach was sprinkled with whites. Half an hour later, we were alone. I had naively assumed that beaches were for swimming regardless of skin color. I had just completed my undergraduate work in psychology and philosophy and was committed in an abstract way to respecting the African-American culture. This was different. This was not theoretical. These people were our primary friends. We played baseball, told stories, and laughed together. Our landlord was the conference moderator. We lived in the African-American community by their invitation, something my faculty at the University where I was completing a masters program in counseling could never understand.

I learned about the experience of the Mennonite church in the south through their eyes. Missionaries had arrived in

North Carolina in the late 1890s from the midwest and with wonderful naivete assumed that if one creates an orphanage it should be available regardless of skin color. Not so, said the town, with rocks through the windows, late night warnings by vigilantes, and cross burnings. So this white couple made it an orphanage for African-Americans from which emerged some of the leadership of the Mennonite churches in the area.

The impact of these experiences on my view of the discipline of psychology and the profession of psychotherapy has been considerable. Even then I studied therapy in the context of a marginal community. My master's thesis (Dueck, 1968) examined self-perceptions among African-American and Caucasian adolescents controlling for social class. As might be predicted, the scores on self-esteem for the Caucasians were higher. The research and experience impressed indelibly on me the connection between social and personal issues. Psychology must deal with the ethical issues of liberation and freedom. Therapy must have something to do with freeing people to experience the new. The biblical narrative describes God as one who frees the oppressed, gives sight to the blind, and creates a liberated people. Given the plight of African-American people, it is obvious that the reign of God has not come in fullness in this nation.

Culture: Recognizing My Ethnic Story

It was not until I returned to Tabor College in 1974 that I began serious work at the dialogue between Christianity and psychology. I discovered at a much more existential level the Anabaptist heritage I had learned about in Sunday school and Bible college. I began to see its relevance to the professional world (Dueck, 1982). That heritage focused on a radical discipleship ethic, a commitment to accountable Christian community, and a critique of society. I spent considerable time thinking about the connection between my Anabaptist heritage and my psychological interests (Klassen and Dueck, 1976). Instead of integration, segregation set in. I was increasingly aware of the larger social world I was living in. Civil religion, nuclearism, individualism, and sexism were part of North American society. How could the discipline of psychology or mental health professionals avoid the influence of Western culture? How does one deal with issues of justice (Dueck, 1976)?

In the summer of 1983 I participated in a postgraduate seminar at Yale University in psychology of religion. We were asked to introduce ourselves at length. One person mentioned where studies and degrees were completed and talked of research interests. Others mentioned reasons for participating in the seminar and their personal hopes for our summer together. I did something I had not done before: I told my Mennonite story.

During my graduate training I had been reticent about my Mennonite faith heritage and its connection to the research I was conducting. I grew up in an ethnic Mennonite home. I sensed that as an ethnoreligious group we had never really made it into contemporary society, given our ethnic foods, use of the German language, and isolated ethnic enclaves. The sense of ethnic embarrassment followed me through college and graduate school. That summer at Yale I decided to risk it.

My story, I began, is one that has its roots in the left wing of the Reformation, develops in the Netherlands in the seventeenth century, winds through Poland and South Russia in the eighteenth and nineteenth centuries, and continues through Canada and the United States into the present century. As I wandered through the eras I mentioned events that shaped my self-perceptions: the importance of the call to follow Christ; persecution by the magisterial reformers for refusing to baptize infants; small house churches that called individual Christians into communal accountability; long migrations replete with illness, privation, and death; my own growing up in an ethnic Mennonite community in Canada; and some of my experiences in the church.

In their desire to follow Christ in obedience, the sixteenth-century Anabaptists gave public expression to their commitment in adult baptism. The state cannot dictate to the church on matters that were her concern. The state, however, found such actions a threat and so the Anabaptists (rebaptizers) were drowned, burned, or killed. That story I have heard told and retold. The implicit message was always that being a disciple of Christ *(Nachfolge Christi)* affects all of life. We are to live a life of quiet resignation to God's will *(Gelassenheit)*. My story invites me not to coerce—choices are to be voluntary (contra Constantinianism). It reinforced the fact that the freedom to express my faith requires that I grant others their freedom as well. The Christian life is communal *(Gemeinschaft)*.

What happened thereafter in that summer seminar I had never experienced before. Often during a discussion of Freud, Jung, or William James, one of the participants in the seminar would turn to me and ask how I viewed the issue given my Mennonite story. My colleagues helped me to flesh out the implications of my own particular understanding of the Christian story for how one constructs an ethical psychology. I have come to the point where I am not embarrassed about my ethnoreligious story. In fact, I see it as a gift. It is my story, and in ways I sometimes hardly realize, it shapes my theory, research, and therapy. I did not create it. My Mennonite story does not begin with my birth. I am a part of a particular people and a global community, the Mennonite community and the worldwide Christian and human community. My ethnoreligious story is not just my own personal conscious history, it has increasingly larger contexts: the German-speaking Mennonite community (several decades ago), North American culture, migrations from the "old world," the left wing of the Protestant Reformation, the Constantinian and medieval Catholic church, and before that the Greco-Roman and Judeo-Christian heritage. I realize my story is, of course, only one version of that larger particular story of the Reign of God, one instrument in that grander orchestra. On the other hand, being ethnic is a particularity that is affirmed by the fact that God came to a Middle Eastern tribe through whom to speak to the world.

Community: On Becoming More Communal

After four years of undergraduate teaching (1974–78), I was burned out. We had an invitation to teach at Fresno Pacific College, had accepted, but were not ready. So, in the year between teaching in Kansas and moving to the west coast where I would spend five (1979–84) wonderful years teaching at Fresno Pacific College, our family spent a sabbatical in Elkhart, Indiana. I taught part time at Goshen College and attended theology classes at the Associated Mennonite Biblical Seminaries and the University of Notre Dame. These were formative times in shaping my theology. At the level of the heart, however, it was while living with the Fellowship of Hope that personal renewal occurred. I had also wondered what healing would be like in a communal context. We had begun to wonder what the church would look like if it took accountability and body life more seriously. The Fellowship of Hope is an intentional Christian community. It was begun by four seminary families in the early 1970s. They were committed to a vision of the church as a community. They were willing to assume liability for each other. This meant emotional, spiritual, and financial support. They chose to live together in a large frame house in one of Elkhart's transitional neighborhoods. Living arrangements included single family dwellings and households of singles and couples. Economic arrangements then included a common fund and independent family accounts.

Of particular interest to me was their common life. Every Thursday supper was eaten together, a common meal. Often the meal was followed with games, storytelling, and singing. The meals were very simple and nutritious. Sunday evening the community broke into smaller groups of ten or so for discernment and accountability: courtship was discussed, new business ventures were considered, parents were supported, personal difficulties or conflicts with others in the community were worked on. The community attracted profoundly broken people. A family of eight came to the community in need of help. The father was unable to support the entire family. Family life was absolutely chaotic. One of the elders spent significant time with the parents teaching them a system of budgeting. In the small groups we discussed parenting styles. Other individuals assisted in the parenting process by taking the children separately on excursions. When we left they had been there six years, the father had deserted the family, but the mother was developing a sense of responsibility.

A pregnant fifteen-year-old prostitute came for help. She had no medical insurance. The community paid for it even though they themselves had no medical insurance. After giving up the baby for adoption, she left. A year later she came back, again pregnant. The community helped her once more. Again she gave up the child for adoption and left. The fall we arrived she again arrived pregnant. This time she stayed. She lived with one of the church families. She was unable to cook for herself. They taught her. She became angry when the child cried. The family taught her how to care for the child and to

respond with patience. She began attending church services
and common meal. The child was slowly becoming her own. It
was a moment of incredible rejoicing for the entire community
when she became a Christian and was baptized. But it was
equally sad when several months later she again left.

For several years I had wondered what a healing community
would look like. It was clear that individual families would not
have been able to respond to the young woman's needs had not
the community supported them with financial and emotional
relief. As I have reflected on this experience, it has become
clearer to me that healing always has a communal context and
that the quality of my work as a therapist is in part dependent
on the quality of the community I or my counselees share. It
was Bonhoeffer's (1965) book, *Life Together,* that deeply moved
me during those days. The Fellowship of Hope was making an
attempt to live out their spirituality with clear corporate commitments. This is not the only model of a communal
Christianity, but it does set a contrast to rampant privatistic
Christianity. The modern world—and particularly Western culture—values independence, individual uniqueness, and personal actualization. It is particularly the middle-class male
who sees accountability as meddling and community as oppressive. Christians live in this same world, only they often tend to
bless their individualism with the label of spirituality. In individualistic societies, spirituality is private and personal. How
I live my life is between God and me. Spirituality then has little to do with ethical accountability.

It was refreshing to be with people who emphasized interdependence, community witness, and personal sacrifice. It should
come as no surprise that over the years I have been fascinated
with social and community psychology, network therapy, and
systems theory. I have taught ethics and personality from a
social-psychological perspective, recognizing the importance of
symbolic interactionism and object relations theory. Teaching
counseling in a seminary is one way I feel I still encourage the
development of a healing context, the church community, for
therapy. The experience at the Fellowship of Hope raised for
me the fundamental question: "Who are my people?" (Dueck,
1981). The fact that I have chosen to teach in a seminary context is clearly influenced by my experience at the Fellowship of
Hope (Dueck, 1987).

Of course I do not know, but I do not think I would have considered twelve years of teaching in Christian higher education (Tabor College, Goshen College, and Fresno Pacific College) after my studies at Stanford if it had not been for the life of another community. This time it was a small Mennonite Brethren congregation in Santa Clara, some fifteen miles from Stanford. Its membership numbered less than a hundred and was not growing very quickly. It was not well known and hardly respected by the large and growing evangelical churches in the Santa Clara valley. It faithfully preached the gospel, sensitively cared for its members, tentatively reached out into the community with a day-care center, and joyfully ate together. In the year before graduation a woman in the congregation asked me about my plans. I wasn't sure. Perhaps I would do research at the University of Illinois where some other colleagues were going. Without hesitation she suggested I consider either staying on as their pastor or joining the Tabor College faculty again. Six months later we were on our way back to Kansas.

Community: My Pastoral Self

Since mother was without resources after my father died, she moved with her young family back to the prairies where all her relatives resided, her biological community. We lived in a small 800-square-foot house with three rooms, a crab apple tree, a plum tree, a gooseberry bush, three elms, and a lilac bush. But our community was as large as the Mennonite neighborhood in North Kildonan, Winnipeg. There was Mr. Dyck who took me fishing. Mr. Jantzen encouraged me to obey my mother, and Mr. Unruh gave me a job mowing his lawn. There was Uncle Abe who taught me to drive a car, line up the cross hairs on my rifle, and took me to the Shrine Circus.

My widowed grandmother was my constant companion the first three years in Winnipeg. While my mother raised two very lively, cantankerous boys, she never did so alone. Mother was never so possessive that others could not correct and love her children. We lived on welfare for several years but had the riches of family and congregation. I remember grocery bags at Christmas from the women's sewing circle, and Mr. Suderman who took us out for a special dinner on Father's Day. These were my mother's friends. They were faithful to a widow.

My personal development very much depended on that community. The church and ethnic Mennonite neighborhood reflected many of the qualities of a healing community and gave me good memories that shape me even today. This was a community that allowed me to exercise my gifts. I preached my first sermon at the age of eighteen. I remember wondering aloud in the sermon why our lily-white congregation was not more multicultural. The pastor, who followed my sermon, tried to contain the fallout. The church and neighborhood gave me male models to serve in my father's place, a sense of belonging to community, a regular rhythm of rituals (Thanksgiving, Christmas, baptism, Easter, foot washing, communion, and of course the Sunday school picnics), a network of friends that stimulated me to growth, a story powerful enough to create a community and capable of healing, a community that had clear limits and let you know the consequences when you failed. It could say "no." It was also a community that could say "yes." In short it was a community of ethical discernment, whether I agreed with their ethic or not. I remember most clearly my mother's love for the church. Once as an idealistic adolescent I was severely criticizing the church. Mother said to me, "Alvin [it was always Alvin when the topic was serious], I happen to love the church." I have learned to love God's people, but a critical perspective is at times needed.

During the 1950s a family moved to Winnipeg from Germany. They lived nearby and my mother cared for them. Being very practical, my mother would send for a repairman if they had problems with the washing machine. When their children ran over to say their mother was crying again, my mother would go over to comfort her. Maybe that is why I have been both a pastor and psychologist over the years.

The biblical theme of God's people is a most meaningful one for me. That it has become so I attribute in part to the experience of peoplehood as a child. When Jesus invites Peter to "Feed my sheep," I understand.

Community: Becoming a Professional

I attended a small rural Bible school after high school and I was confident the school would make a preacher out of me. But the two years away from home gave me the opportunity for the individuation I needed and I charted my own direction. It was here that my interest in psychology was kindled. The instructor was a pastor, not a psychologist, and the text he used in 1961 was already quite outdated. But it was clear that psychology could be a servant of the church and my appetite was whetted. It wasn't long before I wondered, "What has Jesus to do with Freud?" It was here in Bible school that I first met Anne. Anne had a zest for life, self-confidence, and a commitment to the life of the church. We were married in 1965 and my love for the discipline of psychology has never matched the passion and romanticism of our relationship.

Dr. Robson, my next psychology instructor at the University of Winnipeg, modeled for me gentleness and scholarship. My world was opened to the insights of Rogers and Skinner, learning theory, and existentialism. I took enough courses in philosophy to constitute a minor concentration. By the third year I felt I needed to be back in theology: this time at the Mennonite Brethren Bible College in Winnipeg. The next two years I attended the Bible college and the university at the same time, a pattern of tacking back and forth that has followed me through the years. I must confess, I didn't know how to put it together: 1 Corinthians and Oedipal conflict, Old Testament theology and norepinephrine. At that point they simply coexisted without animosity. At times I assumed that being a psychologist was really no different than being a pastor. At other times, I felt pastors would do well to converse with psychologists. At yet other times, the enterprise of therapy seemed little more than a business that reflected American capitalism.

I knew I would eventually complete doctoral studies but did not know when. After two years of teaching undergraduate psychology at Tabor College (1969–1971), I took a three year leave of absence (1971–1974). I applied, was accepted at Stanford University, and received a Canada Council Grant to pay expenses. I was elated (or was it inflated?). Stanford with its ivy-covered walls, tile-covered roofs, arched walkways, Memorial Chapel, and Hoover tower gave the impression of academia at its best. The faculty were world renowned, reported to senate subcommittees, were forever publishing books, and seemed to have an unlimited supply of money available to do research. And I was to be one of their students (more hubris!).

Many of the departments ranked highest in the nation. The university research library boasted a million holdings, and its football team (at that time) had again won the Rose Bowl. And I was going to be a graduate of Stanford University, I hoped. I arrived starry eyed and suffering from a colossal inferiority complex. Starry eyed because this upstart from North Kildonan had made it to graduate school, and depressed because he thought he would never make it through. My fellow students came from Harvard, Princeton, and Yale, while my faculty advisor could never remember where I had completed my masters work. Appropriate deflation!

My world was split. Systematic research or cognition and memory on the one hand (Bower, Karlin, and Dueck, 1975), and being associate pastor at El Camino Bible church. It was the church experience that kept my faith alive. Stanford developed the research skills I have used to help my own denomination reflect on itself, using surveys and analysis (Toews, Konrad, and Dueck, 1986; Enns and Dueck, 1988). But Stanford was and is an institution deeply immersed in the modern world where knowledge is power. There is no question that in the modern world knowledge enables one to predict and control. When I reflect on my spirituality while attending Stanford, it is clear that my professional growth was as much a consequence of my church experience during those years as it was because of graduate school. The church qualified the power of the academic community. Essentially, the discipline of psychology and Christianity remained separate the three years at Stanford. Research and reading psychology on the one hand and pastoral work on the other.

I became increasingly aware in the early 1980s of how religious mental health professionals seemed to outgrow the church (Dueck, 1982). Church was what one did on Sunday. It felt like what is sometimes referred to as being a "Saturday night ethnic": an occasional nostalgia for tradition. The rest of the time the standards, customs, and community of the profession prevailed. The individualism of the profession didn't seem to bother them (Dueck, 1980). That behaviorism might be the incarnation of a technological society went unnoticed. To be a Christian professional meant doing what every other member of the profession was doing, only doing it better or with a fish sign on the Volvo bumper or Choice books in the waiting room. The fees were the same. The clients were the same: middle class, the ones who could pay and whose problems were amenable to the middle-class therapy. The church, it seemed, was irrelevant to the profession. Yes, I probably romanticized the church in those days in my reaction to professionalism. But at the same time the church's vision for a new society and a new person was not getting its due. I struggled with the ethos of professionalism.

In 1984, after teaching in undergraduate departments of psychology for twelve years, our denominational seminary invited me to teach in their counseling program. To prepare marriage and family counselors for work in the church and society was a challenge I could not pass up. My thinking and writing those years focused largely on issues of ethics and therapy (Dueck, 1989; Friesen and Dueck, 1988). That culminated in the presentation of the Integration Lectures at the Graduate School of Psychology at Fuller Theological Seminary in January, 1986. The metaphors that shaped the lectures, and later this book, were the ethical implications of the Reign of God, the responsibility of the church in assisting the professional therapist in ethical issues, and the transformation of the character of the therapist as ethical agent by the larger story of the Reign of God and the involvement in the community of faith (Dueck 1986, 1987a, 1987b, 1988).

Eventually, I realized I needed to be actively engaged in therapy to serve as support for my teaching and reflecting, and so began the process of moving toward licensure. At the encouragement of the seminary and friends I "went with it." I needed to complete 3000 hours of supervised therapy and to pass the state licensing exams. I began the process in 1987 and completed it in 1990.

From 1984 to 1991 I directed the Marriage and Family Counseling program at the Mennonite Brethren Biblical seminary. Students went from our program to Christian counseling centers, pastoral positions, and graduate school. My thinking increasingly moved toward the issues of the family in the modern world (Friesen and Dueck, 1990). I taught a course in ethics and family therapy and wondered again how Judeo-

Christian ethics intersected with the various approaches to family therapy (Dueck, 1989, 1992).

Today, in addition to my teaching and writing, I see a few clients and supervise students. Our clients are largely poor. The clientele reflects Fresno's multicultural diversity. The counseling is very difficult. My close friends have commented on the change. Critique of the profession in the 1970s; immersion in the 1990s. Somewhere in the eighties I had begun to change. I began to see the discipline from a more pragmatic point of view. What's useful, use; what's consistent, apply. Avoid the ideology.

I am grateful for the many models of professionalism that I have encountered over the years. I remember a medical doctor who was not so tied to the profession as to be unable to leave his practice and serve in Cambodia, and whose relationship to patients involved an attempt to treat the whole person, not simply a body or one of its parts. I have business acquaintances who consider profit sharing as a way of creating a sense of community between employees and employers. There is the architect I know who is committed to designing buildings or homes that reflect a concern about energy usage and land consumption. I remember a lawyer, who because of God's particular love for the oppressed, chose to work with the weak and helpless in tenant-landlord disputes. I personally know a number of teachers who teach with low pay in difficult ethnic minority schools. Then there are the psychologists listed in the preface who have significantly impacted me.

There have been times for renewal as a therapist and teacher. In the spring of 1991 I was granted a sabbatical. Three of the months were spent at Heidelberg University in Germany with Dr. Helm Stierlin's team of family therapists. What an experience! I was included in a team that worked with families. I could view any of 2000 videotapes of their work over the past fifteen years. I attended classes, read the family journals in their library, and attended an international conference hosted by Stierlin's group. Perhaps the best surprise was to discover that Stierlin has written a pamphlet (in German) entitled, "The Christians in the World Family," in which he shares his own personal faith. The book uses material from the field of family research and from the Sermon on the Mount to talk about peace in the family and in society.

The Heidelberg experience was incredible. Stierlin's warm invitation to come, the generous invitation to use whatever materials were at hand (books, tapes, files, and actual sessions) was more than I expected. Joachen Schweitzer's warm embrace and offer to work with him as a therapeutic team member was unforgettable. During each counseling session the therapists would take a break to plan with us the direction of the remaining time with the family. The fact that this group read widely in linguistics, sociology, and philosophy, and integrated it into therapy was refreshing. Their awareness of the discussions of postmodernity was encouraging. I found myself intrigued by their approach to circular questioning, use of pauses for planning interventions, and their use of metaphor and narrative in therapy.

We lived a half-hour drive away in a small hamlet, Frankenthal. Here a congregation of Russian-Mennonite emigres lived and worshipped. We lived in the home of one of the immigrant families. Their congregational Bible study was most interesting. They selected a text in advance and thus everyone would know which text would be discussed. Young and old attended. The church opened the meeting for everyone to participate. Some had prepared a mini exegesis and shared it. Others responded spontaneously. A variety of perspectives were presented. Young people felt free to present. The church was otherwise rather hierarchical, but in this respect they were very communal. It was a wonderful moment when the moderator said: "Let the church speak," and then sat down and did not say another word until the closing.

What a contrast between Frankenthal and Heidelberg. It felt like Santa Clara and Stanford all over again. Frankenthal represented for me all that is old world, conservative faith. The German spoken was not as elegant, the faith was very simple and somewhat ethnocentric. Heidelberg was cosmopolitan, secular, sophisticated, and complex. Every day I moved between these two worlds. I was clearly at home and loved in the Frankenthal community. In the Heidelberg community I was appreciated for my analysis of family therapy.

This then is my more professional self. I have slowly come to see my work as a vocation. It has a context. That context I want to be the Reign of God. What has changed over the years is a better discernment of when my work is a reflection of modernity and/or a reflection of the Reign of God.

Self: On Developing Masculine Character

One dimension in my journey toward greater wholeness and character involves my masculinity. My maternal and paternal grandparents lived in the Ukraine. But with the Russian revolution and turmoil of the 1920s they emigrated to Canada. It is no surprise that I still have dreams with a cast of Russian revolutionaries! I come from two generations of widows: first my maternal grandmother and then my mother. Grandfather died shortly after arriving in Canada. My father drowned in the Pacific Ocean in a fishing accident when I was two; my mother was pregnant with my brother. It has been interesting to learn of my own father. In his youth he was a creative story-teller for his younger brothers, weaving tales of mystery and intrigue. He was a risk taker. He swam the Dnieper River with inflated wet pillow cases as ballast. When the sun dried them and the air escaped, he swam back to shore. When the Dueck family came to Canada in the 1920s and lived in a small Mennonite town, my father found both his father and the community too restrictive. And so my father traveled the country in railway cars and played fiddle at hoedowns in order to stay alive. In his late twenties, father had a significant religious awakening and then attended a Bible school. He later worked in an auto paint shop, but for health reasons a doctor recommended he not continue. To make extra money he fished. My parents had been living cozily in a houseboat under Second Narrows Bridge in Vancouver, British Columbia. One July day in 1945, he went fishing with another man and they never returned. Two weeks later my father's body washed up on the shore of Vancouver Island.

I have had to learn how to deal with the aftereffects of growing up in a single parent family and living without a father figure. I have had a number of individuals who were male models for me. My father's youngest brother symbolized spontaneity and intellectual curiosity. He was inventive and creative. Though the youngest of the siblings he was quite willing to disagree with the others and chart his own course. He was the first to leave the home town of Winnipeg and become active in the Charismatic movement.

The absence of a father in my childhood created a void. I had never thought of my father's absence as a wound. I do now. I see now what I have missed. Moral character requires strength. Mother tried to model strength and gentleness, but I needed to see it in men. A friend once told me that it was a wound that would never go away. When I protested, he said that, though a tree is wounded, the wound remains and the bark grows around the wound. The wound is also a gift when it doesn't determine my responses. It may in fact be connected to what gifts I possess. I think it has kept alive in me the importance of tenderness, a tenderness that has also been the reason for a lack, at times, of confidence. With many of my contemporaries I wrestle with what it means to be male. I have had to deal with patriarchal institutions, dogmatic theologies, and ideological psychologies. The metaphor of God as father has been helpful. It has qualified the power of institutions, theologies, and ideologies on the one hand, and pointed to the gentleness of a father on the other. I understand that God as father is more meaningful to me than for someone whose father has been abusive. I pray "Abba Father" with joy.

Self: A Matter of Heart

Ethics without heart easily reduces to legalism and raw duty. Over the years I have had to discover a religion of the heart that leads to character. Perhaps what has created the most change in me over the past decade is a consequence of listening to the suffering of the persons I see as clients. I have had to take stock of my own heart. Some twenty years of scholarship take their toll. I began wondering what the impact might be on my therapy, not to mention on my own spiritual life. Let me share a dream I had that forced me to take more seriously the condition of my own heart.

> I am taking our son Kevin to the hospital. He is around twelve at the time and the event takes place somewhere in Canada. I cannot remember the reason for hospitalization, but I do remembers boxes in the aisles which I have to avoid. While I am waiting for the examination to end, I hear over the intercom

that Kevin is being rushed into emergency surgery. I next remember standing in the surgery room watching as they wheel Kevin in. He is lying on a gurney with doctors hovering over him. The surgeon pours a thick red liquid on him that resembles blood. It gathers on the side. He then takes a knife and begins to cut once lengthwise and once crosswise. I begin to cry uncontrollably, am discovered, and ushered out into the lobby where many relatives have gathered.

I did not sleep well the rest of that night. I took this dream as a warning. It was not my son's heart that needed radical surgery, it was my own. I needed the blood that gives life to my body and so the surgeon had to add it. What I needed was open heart surgery. Why? Many reasons. The fundamentalist religion I grew up with as a child induced much guilt and fear of the afterlife. It was a harsh religion, and it had a way of silencing the whisperings of a young and sensitive heart. The warm piety I experienced in high school and Bible school was formative. But by the time I finished graduate school it seemed disconnected from the larger world. When I encountered the Anabaptist emphasis on ethics and community, I found a different kind of piety.

But in all that, I had forgotten the God who is within: the God who has taken on human form and experience (John 1). For too many years I had been reading, writing, and teaching, not listening to my heart, not listening to the Spirit of God. I am not sure I trusted a faith that follows a grammar of the heart. Of course, it was not a matter of returning or recovering my adolescent piety; I had to encounter God anew given my present stage.

So what is this religion of the heart? Well, first, I think that we are so constituted that there is in our hearts a hunger for God's presence. In the words of Augustine, "Our hearts are restless until they find their rest in thee." I think deep within our souls we are invited to recognize a Presence. The God of Sarah and Mary comes to us not only in the gathered community, but also alone, in our hearts. And what does it mean for me? That I learn to wait for the God who seeks me. If with all my heart I seek God, I discover that I find God's presence in my soul when I create room in my psyche. It comes as I write in my journal, when I am ruthlessly honest with myself about my motives, my hopes, and my fears. It comes when I recognize my injuries and wounds. Our hearts are filled with a mixture of primary metaphors, dreams, stories, images that give meaning to our lives. These I want to be enriched, changed, and affirmed by the presence of God.

Slowly I have begun to understand when I need to separate my inner promptings and God's Spirit, when to say "this is my dream and it is the presence of God; and it is good." Sometimes it has meant for me to be spontaneous, and sometimes measured. In the Christmas season I am often moved by the example of Mary, the mother of Jesus. Mary is one who saw with her heart. She is silent and reflective. The angel appears to Joseph, as one would expect in a patriarchal society. But it is Mary's heart that breaks forth in song. It appears that there had been some years of preparation of heart. After the shepherds left "Mary treasured up all these things and pondered them in her heart" (Luke 2:19).

Self: Ethics as Iconography

My faith is more than firmly held intellectual convictions. It has been influenced by the realization that, for many, faith is shaped by the senses: seeing, hearing, taste, and touch. Orthodox Christians have reminded me of this simple fact. The Soviet Orthodox Church, which rose up before me in Kiev one October morning, was an imposing structure. The columns painted white, the walls blue. The golden onion domes glinted in the morning sun. As I entered, the words of a friend familiar with Orthodoxy came back to me: "To enter the church is always to enter worship service already in progress." At this very moment a heavenly host of angels and departed saints praise God. I was told the praise and beauty of the heavenly scene is to be replicated in the church. The beauty of the surroundings are visual reflections of heavenly beauty. They are created to image forth the beauty of truth.

As I entered, the smell of incense, the murmur of prayer, and the smell of human bodies greeted me. A choir nestled somewhere in the many naves of the cathedral responded to the sonorous bass of the priest. The church was lit only by ubiquitous candles, their sputtering and crackling seemed to merge with the litany. All around me were diminutive elderly women with bowed heads. I stood quietly, hands behind me. I felt a touch on my hands. I turned to hear one of these babushka-covered women speaking to me in Russian and pointing to my hands. I used up my entire Russian vocabulary telling her I didn't understand. I thought perhaps my posture was less than reverent and so I folded my hands in front of me. The babushka nodded approval. As in other orthodox cathedrals I had seen, the front was covered with five rows of icons: paintings of God the Father, of Jesus, the Holy Sprit, the patron saint of the cathedral, the disciples, and of the great church fathers. We worshipped under their silent gaze.

I wondered about the superficiality of our national icons. I wondered where were the powerful images in my austere Anabaptist tradition? I realized that in my tradition I am called to be an icon, a living icon that illustrates an ethic. After all, we are created in the image of God. We are icons that, with care, may show forth the majesty of God. By who we become, we reflect the beauty of the incarnated Christ. By the sacrifice willingly made, by the conflict resolved, by the voice raised for the voiceless, we become icons.

As I stood there in that cavernous cathedral, from out of the crannies of my mind I heard an old script. "Perhaps word and text are much more important." "No," I said to myself, "like the Magi of old these Christians bring to worship gold, frankincense, and myrrh." Here is a faith that survived Ivan the Terrible and Stalinism. These Eastern Christians understand the connection between incarnation and beauty, theological dyslexia and creativity. Deep down, though, I am still an Anabaptist. The icons that move me most are human: those whose character reflect the character of their God in kindness, love, courage, and wisdom.

Self: Character and Symbol

I did not grow up in a particularly artistic ethos in the 1950s. There was no Picasso print hanging on our walls. I heard neither Beethoven nor Mozart. Rilke and Dostoyevsky were unknowns. And so the journey to Rome at the end of the sabbatical in Germany changed something within me.

Mother cleaned homes, she did not paint landscapes. But what was absent she made up for by taking us to the Winnipeg music festival and paying for years of violin and piano lessons.

Mother's idea of beauty was a well-cleaned home and a pure heart.

St. Peter's was immense, beautiful, awesome. I stood and reflected on the Pieta, the marble sculpture by Michelangelo of the Mother of Jesus with the dead Jesus draped across her lap. The sense of suffering and impotence in the face of death was overwhelming. I gazed at the ceiling of the Sistine Chapel ablaze with colors with scene after scene of the biblical story. The Chapel and its incredible churchly art is what the Protestants paid for their separation: a sense of symbol.

And I was not alone. There were hundreds of people around me viewing the same story. And for the past four hundred years or so people have viewed these same images. I did not feel this beauty was the exclusive property of Roman Catholicism. I felt it was ours: it was catholic. What intrigued me was that Michelangelo's work touched the hearts of many people with divergent beliefs, cultures, and lifestyles. He evoked in me the feelings that go with the universal themes of suffering in all of us. In the midst of the incredible pluralism of modernity there is still clearly some consensus that draws people into religious circles. Again I realized the importance of feeding my soul, of taking the time to soak up the beauty of someone else's spiritual labor. It has a way of putting into perspective what is secondary or trivial. As a result of my experience in Rome, I have begun to wonder what would happen if I saw my work as teacher and therapist as one of creating beauty. Not just artists are invited to do that.

These then are my more personal explorations into the meaning of character. Without question my soul is a work in progress. This autobiographical chapter is also an attempt to understand my story as a part of the larger narrative of the Reign of God and my Mennonite heritage. I see more now than I did when I first experienced what I have described. Even in the writing of my story I would seek first the Reign of God. Its language is my primary language; its plot is to become my primary plot. Its central character I seek to imitate and assimilate.

Bibliography

American Psychological Association. (1992). Ethical Principles of Psychologists. *American Psychologist* 47:1597–1611.

Adams, R. (1972). *Watership Down.* New York: Avon Books.

Albee, G. (1977). The Protestant Ethic, Sex, and Psychotherapy. *American Psychologist* 32:150–61.

———. (1977). Does Including Psychotherapy in Health Insurance Represent a Subsidy to the Rich from the Poor? *American Psychologist* 32:719–21.

Alves, R. (1977). Personal Wholeness and Political Creativity: The Theology of Liberation and Pastoral Care. *Pastoral Psychology* 26:124–36.

Ashbrook, J. B. (1987). *On Being a Pioneer.* Paper given at American Association of Pastoral Counselors, New Orleans.

Augsburger, D. (1986). *Pastoral Counseling Across Cultures.* Philadelphia: Westminster.

Back, K. W. (1978). An Ethical Critique of Encounter Groups. In *Ethics of Social Intervention,* ed. G. Bermant, H. Kelman, and D. Warrick. New York: Halstead.

Banks, R. (1980). *Paul's Idea of Community: The Early House Churches in Their Historical Setting.* Grand Rapids, MI: Eerdmans.

———. (1983). The Early Church as a Caring Community. *Evangelical Review of Theology* 7:310–27.

———. (1987). *All the Business of Life: Bringing Theology Down to Earth.* Sutherland: Albatross Books.

243

Barbour, I. G. (1974). *Myths, Models, and Paradigms.* New York: Harper & Row.

Barrett, W. (1986). *Death of the Soul.* New York: Anchor.

Barth, K. (1960). *Church Dogmatics.* III/2, Edinburgh, England: T & T Clark.

Barth, M. (1959). Christ and Law. *Oklahoma Law Review* 12:67–85.

Bateson, G. (1972). *Steps to an Ecology of Mind.* New York: Ballantine.

———. (1979). *Mind and Nature: A Necessary Unity.* New York: E. P. Dutton.

Bellah, R., R. Madsen, W. Sullivan, A. Swidler, and S. Tipton. (1985). *Habits of the Heart: Individualism and Commitment in American Life.* Berkeley: University of California.

Berger, P., ed. (1977). *Facing up to Modernity: Excursion in Society, Politics and Religion.* New York: Random House.

Berger, P. L. and T. Luckmann. (1966). *The Social Construction of Reality: A Treatise in the Sociology of Knowledge.* Garden City, NY: Doubleday.

Berger, P. L., B. Berger, and H. Keller. (1973). *The Homeless Mind: Modernization and Consciousness.* New York: Random House.

Berkhof, H. (1962). *Christ and the Powers.* Trans. J. H. Yoder. Scottdale, PA: Herald.

Bettelheim, B. (1977). *The Uses of Enchantment.* New York: Vintage Books.

Bloom, Fred. (1977). Psychotherapy and Moral Culture: A Psychiatrist's Field Report. *Yale Review* 66:321–46.

Bly, Robert. (1990). *Iron John.* Reading, MA: Addison Wesley.

Bonhoeffer, D. (1963). *Sanctorum Communio.* London: Collins.

———. (1965). *Life Together.* London: SCM Press.

———. (1985). *Spiritual Care.* Trans. J. C. Rochelle. Philadelphia: Fortress.

Borg, Marcus. (1984). *Conflict, Holiness and Politics in the Teachings of Jesus.* Toronto: Edwin Mellen.

———. (1988). *Jesus: A New Vision.* San Francisco: Harper & Row.

Bower, Gordon, M. Karlin, and A. Dueck. (1975). Comprehension and Memory for Pictures. *Memory and Cognition* 3:216–20.

Brandt, L. (1970). American Psychology. *American Psychologist* 25:1091–94.

Browning, Don S. (1966). *Atonement and Psychotherapy.* Philadelphia: Westminster.

———. (1976). *Moral Context of Pastoral Care.* Philadelphia: Westminster.

———. (1983a). *Religious Ethics and Pastoral Care.* Philadelphia: Fortress.

———. ed. (1983b). *Practical Theology.* Philadelphia: Westminster.

———. (1988a). The Pastoral Counselor as Ethicist: What Difference Do We Make? *The Journal of Pastoral Care* 42:283–98.

Brueggemann, W. (1979). Covenanting as Human Vocation. *Interpretation* 33:115–29.

Bryant, D., J. Kessler, and L. Shirar. (1992). *The Family Inside: Working with the Multiple.* New York: W. W. Norton.

Buber, M. (1958). *I and Thou.* Trans R. Smith. New York: Charles Scribner's.

———. (1958). *Tales of Hassidic Masters.* New York, NY: Schocken Books.

———. (1965). *Between Man and Man.* New York: Macmillan.

———. (1965). *The Knowledge of Man: A Philosophy of the Interhuman.* New York: Harper & Row.

Buss, A. R. (1975). The Emerging Field of Sociology of Psychological Knowledge. *American Psychologist* 30:998–1002.

———. ed. (1979). *Psychology in Social Context.* New York: Irvington.

Cashdan, Sheldon. (1988). *Object Relations Therapy: Using the Relationship.* New York: Norton.

Corey, G., M. Schneider, and P. Callanan. (1984). *Issues and Ethics in the Helping Professions.* Monterey, CA: Brooks/Cole Publishing Co.

Cox, D. (1959). *Jung and Saint Paul.* New York: Association.

Crossan, John Dominic. (1975). *The Dark Interval: Towards a Theology of Story.* Niles, IL: Argus Communication.

Crites, S. (1971). The Narrative Quality of Experience. *Journal of the American Academy of Religion* 39:291–311.

Davies, W. D. (1958). *Paul and Rabbinic Judaism.* London.

De Tocqueville, A. (1956). *Democracy in America.* New York: Mentor.

Dueck, A. (1968). *The Relationship of Self-Esteem in Negro and White Adolescents to Perception of Others.* Unpublished master's thesis.

———. (1976). Education for Justice. *Direction* 5:14–22.

———. (1979). *Perception of Order in Scrambled Text.* Unpublished doctoral thesis, Stanford University.

———. (1980). Contexts of Conversion. *Direction* 9:10–15.

———. (1981). Who Are My People? In *Perils of Professionalism.* Eds. D. Kraybill and P. Good. Scottdale, PA: Herald.

———. (1982). Contexts of Professionalism. Paper presented at the Annual Mennonite Graduate Seminar, Manhattan, Kansas. August.

———. (1982). Prolegomena to Mennonite Approaches in Mental Health Services. *Mennonite Quarterly Review* 56:45–65.

———. (1983). A Nuclear Blast Can Ruin Your Whole Day. Forum chaired at Christian Association of Psychological Studies.

———. (1985). North American Psychology: Gospel of Modernity. *Conrad Grebel Review* 3:165–78.

———. (1986). Sectarian Pastoral Care. In *Dictionary of Pastoral Care and Pastoral Counseling.* Ed. Rodney J. Hunter. Nashville: Abingdon.

———. (1987a). Ethical Contexts of Healing: Ecclesia and Praxis. *Pastoral Psychology* 36:49–60.

———. (1987b). Ethical Contexts of Healing: Peoplehood and Righteousness. *Pastoral Psychology* 35:239–53.

———. (1987c). Pastoral Caregivers. In *Deacons and the Church: A Brethren/Mennonite Project.* Ed. Jay Gibble. Elgin.

———. (1988a). Ethical Contexts of Healing: Character and Ritual. *Pastoral Psychology* 36:69–83.

———. (1988b). Psychology and Mennonite Self-Understanding. In *Mennonite Identity.* Eds. C. Redekop and S. Steiner. New York: University of America Press, 203–24.

———. (1989). On Living in Athens: Models of Relating Psychology, Church and Culture. *Journal of Christianity and Psychology* 8:5–18.

———. (1989). Story, Community and Ritual: Anabaptist Themes and Mental Health. *Mennonite Quarterly Review* 63:77–91.

———. (1992). Congregational Care Needs and Resources Study: A Summary. *Direction* 21:26–41.

———. (1992). Metaphors, Models, Paradigms and Stories in Family Therapy. In *Family Therapy: Christian Perspectives.* Ed. Hendrika Vande Kemp. Grand Rapids, MI: Baker.

———. (1992). The Church as a Healing Community. *Builder* 1–9.

Durkheim, E. (1951). *Suicide.* Glencoe, IL: Free Press.

Durnbaugh, D. (1968). *The Believers Church.* New York: Macmillan.

Dykstra, C. (1981). *Vision and Character: A Christian Educator's Alternative to Kohlberg.* Ramsey, NJ: Paulist Press.

Ebersole, A. (1961). *A Critical Comparison of the Anabaptist View of the Church and the Therapeutic Community in Contemporary Psychiatric Practice.* Unpublished master's thesis, University of Chicago.

Eliot, T. S. (1940). *Christianity and Culture.* New York: Harcourt Brace Jovanovich.

Elizur, J. and S. Minuchin. (1989). *Institutionalizing Madness: Families, Therapy, and Society.* New York: Basic.

Ellul, J. (1964). *The Technological Society.* New York: Vintage.

———. (1967). *The Presence of the Kingdom.* New York: Seabury.

———. (1974). Work and Calling. In *Callings.* Eds. J. Y. Holloway and W. D. Campbell. New York: Paulist, 18–44.

———. (1978). *The Betrayal of the West.* New York: Seabury.

Enns, R. and A. Dueck. (1988). Mennonite Brethren in Three Countries: Comparative Profiles of an Ethno Religious Tradition. *Direction* 17:30–59.

Erikson, E. (1953). *Childhood and Society.* New York: Norton.

Estes, C. P. (1992). *Women Who Run with the Wolves.* New York: Ballantine.

Farnsworth, K. (1985). *Wholehearted Integration: Harmonizing Psychology and Christianity through Word and Deed.* Grand Rapids, MI: Baker.

Fellner, C. (1976). The Use of Teaching Stories in Conjoint Family Therapy. *Family Process* 15:428ff.

Fenn, Richard K. (1978). *Toward a Theory of Secularization.*

Society for the Scientific Study of Religion Monograph Series #1.

Foster, R. (1978). *Celebration of Discipline*. New York: Harper & Row.

———. (1985). *Money, Sex and Power*. New York: Harper & Row.

Frank, J. D. (1963). *Persuasion and Healing: A Comparative Study of Psychotherapy*. New York: Schocken.

Frankl, V. (1963). *Man's Search for Meaning*. New York: Pocket Books.

Frei, H. (1982). *The Eclipse of Biblical Narrative: A Critical Introduction*. Nashville: Abingdon.

Freud, S. (1927/1961). *The Future of an Illusion*. Ed. and trans. J. Stachey. New York: Norton.

———. (1936/1961). *Civilization and its Discontents*. Trans. J. Strachey. New York: Norton.

Friesen, W. and A. Dueck. (1988). Whatever happened to Law? *Journal of Psychology and Christianity* 7:13–22.

Gardner, R. (1971). *Therapeutic Communication with Children: The Mutual Storytelling Technique*. New York: Science House.

Gazzaniga, M. (1985). *The Social Brain*. New York: Basic.

Geertz, C. (1973). *The Interpretation of Cultures*. New York: Basic.

Gergen, K. J. (1973). Social Psychology as History. *Journal of Personality and Social Psychology* 26:309–20.

———. (1982). *Transformation in Social Knowledge*. New York: Springer-Verlag.

———. (1991). *The Saturated Self.* New York: Basic.

Gerkin, C. (1984). *The Living Human Document: Revisioning Pastoral Counseling in a Hermeneutical Mode*. Nashville: Abingdon.

———. (1986). *Widening the Horizons: Pastoral Responses to a Fragmented Society*. Philadelphia: Westminster.

Gilligan, C. A. (1981). *In a Different Voice*. Cambridge, MA: Harvard University Press.

Gish, A. (1979). *Living in Christian Community*. Scottdale, PA: Herald.

Goldberg, M. (1982). *Theology and Narrative: A Critical Introduction*. Nashville: Abingdon.

Goldstein, A. P. (1973). *Structured Learning Therapy: Toward a Psychotherapy for the Poor.* New York: Academic Press.

Good, P. and D. Kraybill. (1982). *Perils of Professionalism.* Scottdale, PA: Herald.

Goode, William J. (1957). Community Within a Community: The Professions. *American Sociological Review* 22:194–200.

Goodwin, R. N. (1974). Reflections: The American Condition. *New Yorker* 35–60.

Gordon, D. (1978). *Therapeutic Metaphors.* Cupertino, CA: Metakin.

Greenberg, J. R. and S. Mitchell. (1983). *Object Relations in Psychoanalytic Theory.* Cambridge, MA: Harvard University Press.

Groome, T. (1980). *Christian Religious Education.* San Francisco: Harper & Row.

Gross, M. L. (1978). *The Psychological Society.* New York: Random House.

Guggenbuehl-Craig, A. (1986). *Power in the Helping Professions.* Dallas, TX: Spring.

Gursslin, O. R., R. G. Hunt, and J. L. Roach. (1959–1960). Social Class and the Mental Health Movement. *Social Problems* 7:210–18.

Gurvitsch, G. (1971). *The Social Frameworks of Knowledge.* New York: Harper & Row.

Gustafson, J. (1968). *Christ and the Moral Life.* New York: Harper & Row.

———. (1971). *Christian Ethics and the Community.* Philadelphia, PA: Pilgrim Press.

Habermas, J. (1972). *Knowledge and Human Interests.* Boston: Beacon.

Halleck, S. L. (1971). *The Politics of Therapy.* New York: Harper & Row.

———. (1971). Therapy Is the Handmaiden of the Status Quo. *Psychology Today* 25:31–39.

Hallie, P. (1979). *Lest Innocent Blood Be Shed.* New York: Harper & Row.

Hare-Mustin, R. C. (1978). A Feminist Approach to Family Therapy. *Family Process* 17:181–94.

———. (1987). The Problem of Gender in Family Therapy. *Family Process* 26:15–27.

Harré, R. and P. F. Secord. (1972). *The Explanation of Social Behavior*. Oxford, England: Basil Blackwell.

Hauerwas, S. (1974). *Character and the Christian Life: A Study of Theological Ethics*. San Antonio, TX: Trinity University Press.

———. (1974). *Vision and Virtue: Essays in Christian Ethical Reflection*. Notre Dame: Fides Publishers.

———. (1977). *Truthfulness and Tragedy: Further Investigations into Christian Ethics*. Notre Dame: University of Notre Dame Press.

———. (1981). *A Community of Character: Toward a Constructive Christian Social Ethic*. Notre Dame: University of Notre Dame Press.

———. (1983). *The Peaceable Kingdom*. South Bend, IN: Notre Dame Press.

Heschel, A. J. (1965). *Who Is Man?* Stanford, CA: Stanford University Press.

Hillman, J. (1972). *The Myth of Analysis*. Evanston, IL: Northwestern University Press.

———. (1975a). The Fiction of Case History: A Round. In *Religion and Story*. Ed. James B. Wiggins. New York: Harper & Row, 123–74.

———. (1975b). *Loose Ends*. Zurich, Switzerland: Spring Publications.

Hillman, J. and M. Ventura. (1992). *A Hundred Years of Therapy and the World Is Getting Worse*. San Francisco: Harper & Row.

Hobhouse, L. T. (1964). *Liberalism*. New York: Oxford University Press.

Hobson, R. F. (1971). Imagination and Amplification in Psychotherapy. *Journal of Analytical Psychology* 16:122-25.

Hoffman, J. C. (1979). *Ethical Confrontation in Counseling*. Chicago: University of Chicago Press.

———. (1986). *Law, Freedom, and Story: The Role of Narrative in Therapy, Society, and Faith*. Waterloo, ON: Wilfred Laurier University Press.

Hoffman, L. (1981). *Foundations of Family Therapy: A Conceptual Framework for Systems Change*. New York: Basic.

Hogan, R. (1975). Theoretical Egoism and the Problem of Compliance. *American Psychologist* 30:533–40.

Holifield, E. B. (1983). *A History of Pastoral Care in America: From Salvation to Self Realization.* Nashville: Abingdon.

Homans, P. (1974). Carl Rogers's psychology and the theory of mass society. In *Innovations in Client-Centered Therapy.* Eds. D. A. Wexler and L. N. Rice. New York: Wiley.

Hunter, J. D. (1981). *American Evangelicalism: Conservative Religion and the Quandary of Modernity.* New Brunswick: Rutgers University Press.

————. (1982). Subjectivization and the New Evangelical Theodicy. *Journal for the Scientific Study of Religion* 20:39-47.

Illich, I. (1977). *Disabling Professions.* London, England: Marion Boyers.

Jacoby, R. (1975). *Social Amnesia: A Critique of Contemporary Psychology from Adler to Laing.* Boston: Beacon.

Johnson, R. (1986). *Inner Work.* New York: Harper & Row.

Jung, C. G. (1933). *Modern Man in Search of a Soul.* New York: Harcourt Brace Jovanovich.

Keith-Spiegel, P. and G. P. Koocher. (1985). *Ethics in Psychology: Professional Standards and Cases.* Hillsdale: Lawrence Erlbaum.

Kiev, A. (1968). *Curanderismo: Mexican-American Folk Psychiatry.* New York: Free Press.

Klassen, M. and A. Dueck. (1976). Moral Development: Issues and Perspectives. In *Research in Mental Health and Religious Behavior.* Ed. William J. Donaldson, Jr. Atlanta.

Kohlberg, L. (1968). The Child as Moral Philosopher. *Psychology Today* 18–26.

Kottler, J. and W. H. Van Hoose. (1977). *Ethical and Legal Issues in Counseling and Psychotherapy.* San Francisco: Jossey-Bass.

Kraft, C. H. (1979). *Christianity in Culture: A Study in Dynamic Biblical Theologizing in Cross-Cultural Perspective.* Maryknoll: Orbis.

Kraus, Norman. (1974). *The Community of the Spirit.* Grand Rapids, MI: Eerdmans.

Kraybill, D. (1978). *The Upside Kingdom.* Scottdale, PA: Herald.

Kueng, H. (1979). *Freud and the Problem of God.* New Haven, CT: Yale University Press.

Kuhn, T. S. (1970). *The Structure of Scientific Revolutions.* Chicago: University of Chicago Press.

Kurelek, W. (1973). *Someone with Me.* Ithaca: Cornell University Press.

Lasch, C. (1978). *The Culture of Narcissism.* New York: Norton.

Le Joly, E. (1983). *Mother Theresa of Calcutta: A Biography.* San Francisco: Harper & Row.

Lebacqz, Karen. (1985). *Professional Ethics: Power and Paradox.* Nashville: Abingdon.

Lee, J. D. (1984). Counseling and Culture: Some Issues. *The Personnel and Guidance Journal* 63:592–97.

Littell, F. (1952). *The Origins of Sectarian Protestantism: A Study of the Anabaptist View of the Church.* Boston: Staff King.

Locke, J. (1690/1964). *An Essay on Human Understanding.* New York: New American Library.

Loewen, H. (1985). *One Lord, One Church, One Hope, and One God.* Elkhart: Institute for Mennonite Studies.

London, P. (1964). *The Modes and Morals of Psychotherapy* New York: Holt Rinehart and Winston.

Luepnitz, D. A. (1988). *The Family Interpreted: Feminist Theory in Clinical Practice.* New York: Basic.

Lukes, S. (1973). *Individualism.* New York: Harper & Row.

MacIntyre, A. (1966). *A Short History of Ethics.* New York: Macmillan.

———— (1981). *After Virtue.* Notre Dame: University of Notre Dame Press.

Macpherson, C. B. (1962). *The Political Theory of Possessive Individualism: Hobbes to Locke.* London, England: Oxford University Press.

Maloney, N. (1979). Transactional Analysis and Christian Counseling. In *Ways of Christian Counseling,* 35–43. Ed. G. Collins. Irvine: Vision House.

————, ed. (1983). *Wholeness and Holiness: Readings in the Psychology of Mental Health.* Grand Rapids, MI: Baker.

Mannheim, K. (1936). *Ideology and Utopia.* New York: Harcourt, Brace & World.

May, R., C. Rogers, and A. Maslow. (1986). *Politics and Innocence: A Humanistic Debate.* New York: W. W. Norton.

McClendon, J. W., Jr. (1974). *Biography as Theology: How Life Stories Can Remake Today's Theology.* Nashville: Abingdon.

McLendon, J. (1986). *Systematic Theology: Ethics.* Nashville, Abingdon.

McFague, S. (1975). *Speaking in Parables: A Study of Metaphor and Theology.* Philadelphia: Fortress.

Mead, G. H. (1934). *Mind, Self and Society.* Chicago: University of Chicago Press.

Miguez-Bonino, J. (1975). *Doing Theology in a Revolutionary Situation.* Philadelphia: Fortress.

Moltman, J. (1979). The Diaconal Church in the Context of the Kingdom of God. In *Hope for the Church.* Nashville: Abingdon. 21–36.

Morgan, G. W. (1968). *The Human Predicament.* New York: Dell.

Moscovici, S. (1972). Society and Theory in Social Psychology. In *The Social Context of Psychology: A Critical Assessment.* Eds. J. Israel and H. Taijfel. New York: Academic, 22–43.

Myers, D. G. (1978). *The Human Puzzle: Psychological Research and Christian Belief.* New York: Harper & Row.

Navone, J. J and T. Cooper, (1981). *Tellers of the Word.* New York: Le Jacq Publishing.

Neufeld, V. H. ed. (1983). *If We Can Love: The Mennonite Mental Health Story.* Newton, KS: Faith and Life Press.

Niebuhr, J. R. (1951). *Christ and Culture.* New York: Harper & Row.

———. (1963). *The Responsible Self: An Essay in Christian Moral Philosophy.* New York: Harper & Row.

Nisbet, R. A. (1953). *The Quest for Community.* London, England: Oxford University Press.

O'Connor, E. (1976). *The New Community.* New York: Harper & Row.

———. (1981). *Our Many Selves.* New York: Harper & Row.

Oden, T. C. (1966). *Kerygma and Counseling.* New York: Harper & Row.

Ornstein, R. (1986). *Multiminds: A New Way to Look at Human Behavior.* Boston: Houghton Mifflin.

Ouspensky, P. D. (1949). *In Search of the Miraculous.* New York: Harcourt Brace Jovanovich.

Palmer, P. J. (1988). *The Company of Strangers: Christians and the Renewal of American Public Life.* New York: Crossroad/Continuum.

Peck, M. S. (1978). *The Road Less Traveled: A New Psychology of Love, Traditional Values and Spiritual Growth.* New York: Simon & Schuster.

———. (1987). *The Different Drum: Community-Making and Peace.* New York: Simon & Schuster.

Pepper, S. (1944). *World Hypotheses.* Berkeley: University of California.

Perls, F. (1969). *Gestalt Therapy Verbatim.* New York: Bantam.

Poling, J. N. and D. E. Miller. (1985). *Foundations for a Practical Theology of Ministry.* Nashville: Abingdon.

Pope, K., Tabachnick, and P. Keith-Spiegel. (1987). Ethics of Practice: Beliefs and Behaviors of Psychologists as Therapists. *American Psychologist* 993–1006.

Potok, C. (1972). *My Name is Asher Lev.* Greenwich, CN: Fawcett.

Rappaport, J. (1977). *Community Psychology: Values, Research, Action.* New York: Holt, Rinehart & Winston.

Rieff, P. (1959). *Freud: The Mind of the Moralist.* New York: Doubleday.

———. (1966). *Triumph of the Therapeutic.* New York: Harper & Row.

Riegel, K. F. (1972). Influence of Economic and Political Ideologies on the Development of Developmental Psychology. *Psychological Bulletin* 78:129–41.

Robinson, H. W. (1980). *Corporate Personality in Ancient Israel.* Ed. G. M. Tucker. Philadelphia: Fortress.

Rogers, C. R. (1961). *On Becoming a Person.* Boston: Houghton Mifflin.

Rousseau, J. J. (1954). *The Confessions.* Trans. J. M. Cohen. Baltimore: Penguin.

Sampson, E. E. (1977). Psychology and the American Ideal. *Personality and Social Psychology* 35:767–82.

Sanders, E. P. (1977). *Paul and Palestinian Judaism: A Comparison of Patterns of Religion.* Philadelphia: Fortress.

———. (1985). *Jesus and Judaism.* Philadelphia: Fortress.

Sandford, J. (1970). *The Kingdom Within.* New York: Harper & Row.

Sarason, S. B. (1974). *The Psychological Sense of Community: Prospects for a Community Psychology.* San Francisco, CA: Jossey-Bass.

Schoefield, W. (1964). *The Purchase of Friendship.* Englewood Cliffs, NJ: Prentice Hall.

Schwartz, R. (1987). Our Multiple Selves. *Family Therapy Networker* 11:24–31.

———. (1988a). The Internal Family Systems Model: An Expansion of Systemic Thinking into the Level of Internal Process. *Family Therapy Case Studies* 3:61–66.

———. (1988b). Know Thy Selves. *Family Therapy Networker* 12:21–29.

———. (1988c). Working with Internal and External Families. *Family Relations* 8:22–34.

Shafer, R. (1981). Narration and Psychoanalytic Dialogue. In *On Narrative.* Ed. W. T. Mitchell. Chicago: University of Chicago Press, 25–49.

Shur, M. (1976). *The Awareness Trap.* New York: McGraw Hill.

Skinner, B. F. (1971). *Beyond Freedom and Dignity.* New York: Bantam.

Smith, A. (1981). *The Relational Self: Ethics and Therapy from a Black Church Perspective.* Nashville: Abingdon.

Snyder, H. A. (1991). *Models of the Kingdom.* Nashville: Abingdon.

Spence, D. (1982). *Narrative Truth and Historical Truth.* New York: Norton.

Stendahl, K. (1976). *Paul Among the Jews and Gentiles.* Philadelphia: Westminster.

Stout, J. (1988). *Ethics after Babel.* Boston: Beacon.

Sullivan, H. S. (1947). *Conceptions of Modern Psychiatry.* Washington: William Alanson White Psychiatric Foundation.

Tillich, P. (1964). The Theological Significance of Existentialism and Psychoanalysis. In *Theology of Culture.* New York: Oxford University Press, 112–26.

Tjeltveit, A. (1992). The Psychotherapist as Christian Ethicist: Theology Applied to Practice. *Journal of Psychology and Theology* 8:89–98.

Toennies, F. (1957). *Community and Society.* New York: Harper & Row.

Toews, J. E. (1982). Some Thesis Toward a Theology of Law in the New Testament. Council of Mennonite Seminaries. *Occasional Papers,* 43–64.

Toews, J. B., A. Konrad, and A. Dueck. (1986). Mennonite Brethren Church Membership Profiled: 1972–1982. *Direction* 14:1–89.

Turner, V. (1969). *The Ritual Process*. Ithaca, NY: Cornell University Press.

Tweedie, D. (1961). *Logotherapy and the Christian Faith*. Grand Rapids, MI: Baker.

Unger, R. M. (1975). *Knowledge and Politics*. New York: Free Press.

Vanier, J. (1981). *The Challenge of L'Arche*. Ottawa, ON: Novalis, St. Paul University.

———. (1989). *Community and Growth*. Rev. ed. New York: Paulist.

Vitz, P. C. (1977). *Psychology as Religion: The Cult of Self-Worship*. Grand Rapids, MI: Eerdmans.

Von Bertalanffy, L. (1968). *General Systems Theory*. New York: G. Braziller.

Wallach, M. A. and L. Wallach. (1983). *Psychology's Sanction for Selfishness: The Error of Egoism in Theory and Therapy*. San Francisco: W. H. Freeman.

Watson, J. B. (1913). Psychology as the Behaviorist Views It. *Psychological Review* 20:158–77.

Weber, M. (1930). *Protestant Ethic and the Spirit of Capitalism*. London: Methuen.

Weinstein, F. and G. Platt. (1969). *The Wish to Be Free: Society, Psyche and Value Change*. Berkeley: University of California Press.

Whitlock. (1960). The Structure of Personality in Hebrew Psychology. *Interpretation* 33:3–13.

Wilk, J. (1985). That Reminds Me of a Story. *Family Therapy Networker* 9:49–52.

Wingren, G. (1957). *Luther on Vocation*. Philadelphia: Muhlenberg.

Wink, W. (1984). *Naming the Powers*. Philadelphia: Fortress.

———. (1986). *Unmasking the Powers*. Philadelphia: Fortress.

———. (1992). *Engaging the Powers*. Philadelphia: Fortress.

Wolff, H. W. (1974). *Anthropology of the Old Testament*. Trans. Margaret Kohl. Philadelphia: Fortress.

Wolff, R. P. (1968). *The Poverty of Liberalism*. Boston: Beacon.

Wolterstorff, N. (1983). *Until Justice and Peace Embrace*. Grand Rapids, MI: Eerdmans.

Yoder, J. H. (1960). The Otherness of the Church. *Concern* 8:19–29.

———. (1964). Richard Niebuhr–Christ and Culture: Analysis and Critique. Paper presented to the Student Services Summer Seminar. Elkhart, IN. August.

———. (1972). *The Politics of Jesus.* Philadelphia: Westminster.

———. (1972). *The Original Revolution.* Scottdale, PA: Herald.

Zuinga, R. (1975). The Experimenting Society and Radical Social Reform. *American Psychologist* 30:99–115.

Index